Catalina Rodriguez
Gabriela Cedeño

Level of knowledge of basic and advanced CPR

Catalina Rodriguez
Gabriela Cedeño

Level of knowledge of basic and advanced CPR

ScienciaScripts

Imprint

Any brand names and product names mentioned in this book are subject to trademark, brand or patent protection and are trademarks or registered trademarks of their respective holders. The use of brand names, product names, common names, trade names, product descriptions etc. even without a particular marking in this work is in no way to be construed to mean that such names may be regarded as unrestricted in respect of trademark and brand protection legislation and could thus be used by anyone.

Cover image: www.ingimage.com

This book is a translation from the original published under ISBN 978-620-3-87700-7.

Publisher:
Sciencia Scripts
is a trademark of
Dodo Books Indian Ocean Ltd., member of the OmniScriptum S.R.L Publishing group
str. A.Russo 15, of. 61, Chisinau-2068, Republic of Moldova Europe
Printed at: see last page
ISBN: 978-620-4-16380-2

To God because He has always been with me since I started this beautiful career and has filled me with health and wisdom.

To my parents Oscar Cedeño and Celina Zambrano who have been my fundamental pillars throughout this process, for their advice, love and for never letting me give up. Thanks to them I have accomplished many achievements

My brothers who always encouraged me to keep going and not fall.

To my boyfriend Jorge who has been with me throughout this race supporting me and giving me strength to continue and not give up.

To my parents Alonso Rodríguez and Yolanda Ordoñez for their sacrifice and effort, for giving me a career for our future, for believing in my ability, for always persevering and fulfilling my ideals.

To my beloved son Juan Sebastián Benavides for being my source of motivation and inspiration to better myself every day.

To my siblings Angely Rodriguez and David Rodriguez whose words of encouragement kept me going.

THANK YOU

Mainly to God for allowing me to finish this career, my family who have supported me in all my decisions.

To my teachers who have formed me to be a great doctor.

To all the Doctors, Graduates and Staff of the Sacred Heart of Jesus Hospital, who welcomed us with open arms so that we could do our internships.

Thanks to Dr. Wladimir Albán who guided and advised us in our degree work.

TABLE OF CONTENTS

SUMMARY

Cardiopulmonary resuscitation is defined as a sequential and organized response to cardiac arrest, which includes: recognizing the absence of circulation and respiration, basic life support with chest compressions and ventilations, advanced cardiac life support in which there is definitive control of the airway and rhythm, and treatment after resuscitation. The objective is to determine the knowledge in the management of basic and advanced cardiopulmonary resuscitation in the health personnel of the emergency area in the Hospital Sagrado Corazón de Jesús Quevedo, in the period from August-September 2020.The research was conducted in the service of the emergency area of the hospital Sagrado Corazón de Jesús de Quevedo. The materials used were medical journals, internet access, editorial. The population of health professionals of the Hospital Sagrado Corazón de Jesús of the Emergency Area is 40 people of which we were able to evaluate the 40 people who were available and willing to take the surveys for the research. The results according to the data, we obtained that the level of knowledge about CPR of the health personnel predominates the high level of knowledge with 65%, due to the fact that the greater percentage of the professionals have been trained. The conclusion of our investigation was that the medical professionals who trained by their own means during the last 3 years have a high and medium level of knowledge in equal percentage and a low percentage have not been trained.

Key words: Cardiopulmonary resuscitation, basic life support.

INTRODUCTION

The present research work will deal with the evaluation of the knowledge of basic and advanced cardiopulmonary resuscitation (CPR) in the health personnel of the emergency area. It will be applied to resident physicians and licensed professionals, who are the ones who provide care to people who are in a critical state, for this reason it is essential to have knowledge of the subject. Cardiorespiratory arrest (CRA) is a serious situation that compromises the patient's life. The main cause of death worldwide is coronary heart disease. Every year worldwide, more people die from cardiovascular pathologies than from any other cause. About three quarters of deaths related to heart disease and stroke occur in low- and middle-income countries. (1) In the emergency area of the Sacred Heart of Jesus Hospital, we observe that all types of patients are admitted in critical condition that require very rapid and immediate attention and action by health personnel, thus providing correct basic and advanced cardiopulmonary resuscitation. In order to perform the functions of health personnel correctly, continuous preparation is necessary to provide optimal care in compliance with quality standards, especially in the management of critically ill patients who require basic and advanced CPR intervention, where the health professional must have a scientific basis in the management of techniques, maneuvers and drugs.

According to the experiences of some evaluators of all the CPRs, it is evident that there are problems in the execution by the health professionals who intervene in a CPR, in the great majority of the cases evaluated it has been shown that the health personnel have a lack of knowledge in the use of adequate medication, CPR constitutes a set of standardized maneuvers of sequential development, internationally accepted, whose initial objective is to substitute and then reestablish respiration, circulation and the integrity of the central nervous system. Only if CPR is started within the first few minutes is there a chance of recovery without neurological sequelae" (2). For this reason it is important to determine and characterize the level of knowledge of basic and advanced cardiopulmonary resuscitation of professionals in the emergency area, it is a fundamental piece for the survival of the patient in this critical area, through timely and proper management will be achieved to avoid complications and reduce morbidity and mortality.

It is hoped that this research will contribute to improve or generate strategies in the management of patients with cardiopulmonary arrest, in such a way that CPR maneuvers are strengthened and increased, improving care and avoiding the compromise of the patient's life. In our study, we will identify if the

CPR training included in the knowledge of health care personnel in the emergency area, whether the years of work experience influenced the level of knowledge of CPR, whether the years of work experience did not influence the level of knowledge of CPR, whether the highest percentage of professionals had a low level of knowledge of CPR and whether the highest percentage of professionals did not receive training in CPR. The level of knowledge in variables such as: identification of CPR, chest compressions, ventilation, airway management, ventilation, early fibrillation and administration of compressions will be assessed.

In the city of Quito, the study conducted by Dr. Duchimaza Adriana and Dr. Rodriguez Viviana, it was observed that about 79% of doctors and nurses know the importance of immediate and timely response protocol, 21% have no knowledge, which concluded that the level of knowledge in basic life support (BLS) of doctors and graduates of the hospital is in an acceptable average but not excellent for the care of cardiorespiratory arrest. (3). CRA is an event that occurs frequently in patients admitted to the hospital. It is estimated that approximately 209,000 cases of in-hospital cardiorespiratory arrest occur each year in the United States with a survival rate of 24.8% (2) and 395,000 cases of out-of-hospital cardiorespiratory arrest occur annually with an average survival rate of 12% (4). In Peru, German Aranzábal-Alegría, Araseli Verastegui-Día, a multicenter analytical cross-sectional study was conducted, with a convenience sampling of health professionals from 25 hospitals in Peru, concluded that the level of knowledge was low; this should be considered to generate policies for updating and continuing education, so that health personnel are prepared in theory and practice, thus being able to avoid complications and deaths.

(5) In-hospital cardiopulmonary arrest is preceded by clinical deterioration which can last for hours or days. Protocols have been created that allow us to identify clinical deterioration and intervene in time to prevent CRA. According to several studies, 80% of hospitalized cases of CRA presented alterations in vital signs hours before arrest, therefore, it is possible to intervene before clinical deterioration or cardiorespiratory arrest occurs. (6) CPR protocols include all procedures such as: activation of rescue systems, basic CPR, use of defibrillators, advanced CPR and management of the post-cardiac arrest period in the intensive care unit. Each hospital is responsible for the organization of prevention and rescue systems, ensuring patient safety (7). Immediate initiation of uninterrupted continuous chest compressions and early defibrillation are paramount to success. Speed, efficacy, and correct application of CPR with minute interruptions will result in successful outcomes. (8) The chain of survival plays an important role and consists of 4 links, allowing circulation to be restored and neurological impairment to be avoided. (9) It is of great interest to emphasize that in order for a physician to enter the Ministry of Public Health he/she has a series of responsibilities that must be fulfilled and that are expressed in his/her contract, but it is equally important to be aware that all public servants have the right to be trained by their employer, in this case, the Ministry of Public Health must program and carry out all the courses that are requested so that the servant is updated, and if they do not have personnel that can carry out the training, they can look for an entity outside the public network to do it. "Various articles have dealt with the problem worldwide. Studies have been carried out in England, the United States of America, Japan, New Zealand, Sweden and China, and have reached the same conclusion: there is a lack of training in CPR in

undergraduate medical education programs, recently graduated physicians do not feel comfortable with resuscitation and make serious errors" (10).

The present study was carried out in Ecuador, in the Sacred Heart of Jesus Hospital in the city of Quevedo, and 40 professionals in the emergency area were evaluated. The research work was feasible in the first place by the approval previously granted by the authorities of the University of Guayaquil, and the Directors of the Sacred Heart of Jesus Hospital who authorized the realization of the research. Likewise to the Health Personnel of the Emergency Area. This research work has a quantitative approach, non-experimental design, cross-sectional and observational method. For the collection of data of the present investigation, the survey technique was used and the instrument was a questionnaire, which contains statements that are referred to a series of activities that have been selected in response to the indicators. Once the data were obtained, they were processed by means of statistical packages after the elaboration of the table of codes, assigning to the answer the corresponding value of 1 (correct question) and 0 (incorrect question). All this in order to then be presented in graphs or statistical tables for analysis and interpretation considering the background and theoretical framework, which help us with the explanation of the results and conclusions.

Regarding the level of knowledge of the health professional on the identification of CRA and the conditions for CPR, they presented a high level of knowledge. The relationship between years of experience and level of knowledge showed that there was no statistically significant difference. As in the study carried out in Tanzania, it was observed that the level of knowledge decreases over the years, but this was not significant. (11) In CPR all actions must be timely and effective; personnel with an average level of knowledge do not have the capacity to reverse CPR and can make many errors that can limit recovery, cause sequelae and even lead to death. CRA can happen anywhere, emphasizing that it occurs more frequently in the out-of-hospital setting, for this reason the AHA has developed protocols, which are updated every 5 years and thus provide timely care. It is essential that health personnel be trained in basic and advanced CPR. Resident physicians should have the knowledge and skills to apply CPR techniques, since they are part of the chain of survival.

CHAPTER I

1. THE PROBLEM

1.1. PROBLEM STATEMENT

More people die each year worldwide from cardiovascular disease than from any other cause, with about three-quarters of deaths related to heart disease and stroke occurring in low- and middle-income countries. (1)

Similarly, sudden cardiac arrest is responsible for about 60% of deaths in adult patients with coronary heart disease. (13)

Globally every day more people are exposed to sudden death, by increasing risk factors, according to the World Health Organization (WHO) cardiovascular diseases, cerebrovascular and trauma are very serious public health problems, which will constitute the main causes of sudden or early deaths, unfortunately 98% of all these deaths occur outside hospitals and the vast majority will not receive the necessary help, dying before reaching a hospital center (WHO, 2018).(14).

In the medical emergency area, cardiorespiratory arrest is very frequent and the main treatment in effective cardiopulmonary resuscitation and early defibrillation, due to the high incidence of death from this cause is that the health professional must be prepared for an emergency of this type, so it is very necessary to increase and spread the knowledge of cardiopulmonary resuscitation.

In the emergency area of the Sacred Heart of Jesus Hospital, we observe that all types of patients are admitted in critical condition that require very fast and immediate attention and action by the health personnel, thus providing correct cardiopulmonary resuscitation, both basic and advanced.

The role of both doctors and nurses requires continuous preparation that allows them to provide optimal care in compliance with quality standards, especially in the management of critically ill patients who require basic and advanced cardiopulmonary resuscitation intervention where the health professional must have a scientific foundation in the management of techniques, maneuvers and drugs.

The experiences of some evaluators of all these events (cardiopulmonary resuscitation) showed that there are problems in the execution by health professionals who intervene in a cardiorespiratory arrest, in most of the cases evaluated it has been shown that health personnel have a lack of knowledge in the use of appropriate medications, such as dosage and use of the defibrillator, which can lead to the death of the patient.

Studies of much emphasis carried out in Peru by Reyes, concluded that health personnel in the emergency department of the national maternal-perinatal institution have an average knowledge of basic cardiopulmonary resuscitation. (Reyes Moran, Cybertesis UNMSM, 2016). (15)

In Spain, the study carried out by Peláez showed that knowledge of cardiopulmonary resuscitation is related to work experience, demonstrating that 76.9% have knowledge of CPR. (16)

In Mexico a study conducted by Balcazar showed that 89.34% of the study population of health personnel, demonstrated an unsatisfactory degree of knowledge, thus exposing that there are very serious deficiencies in the knowledge of cardiopulmonary resuscitation, and that the years of experience and ability in resuscitation are not associated with the level of knowledge. (American Heart Association, 2017). (17)

1.2. PROBLEM FORMULATION

To identify the dimension of knowledge about basic and advanced cardiopulmonary resuscitation in the health personnel of the emergency area of the Hospital Sagrado Corazón de Jesús de Quevedo, in the period between August-September 2020.

1.3. DELIMITATION OF THE PROBLEM **Nature of the study:** Observational,

cross-sectional **Field:** Public Health

Area: Emergency

Aspect: Basic and advanced cardiopulmonary resuscitation

Topic: Level of knowledge of basic and advanced cardiopulmonary resuscitation in health personnel.

Spatial delimitation: The research was carried out in the emergency department of the Sagrado Corazón de Jesús Quevedo Hospital.

Time frame: The present study took into account the period August-September 2020.

This research work is a support to determine and characterize the level of knowledge of basic and advanced cardiopulmonary resuscitation of the professionals in the emergency area, it is a fundamental piece for the survival of the patient in this critical area, by means of the opportune and adequate management it will be possible to avoid complications and reduce morbimortality. It will provide information based on scientific evidence and updated on the level of knowledge of basic and advanced CPR of health personnel. It is hoped that this research will contribute to improve or generate strategies in the management of patients with cardiopulmonary arrest, thus strengthening and increasing CPR maneuvers, improving care and avoiding the compromise of the patient's life.

The investigation of this topic is so important since it arises from the interest of knowing and characterizing the level of knowledge of health personnel in the emergency area in relation to basic and advanced cardiopulmonary resuscitation, taking into account that they are the first contact with a vulnerable group such as patients who suffer cardiac arrest and require that the indications and actions be precise.

By applying cardiopulmonary resuscitation maneuvers (CPR) by the people who witnessed the cardiorespiratory arrest increases 7 times the chance of survival. The American Heart Association (AHA) provides updated information through courses on topics of interest such as updated information on arrhythmias and basic and advanced CPR. It is necessary and fundamental that health personnel have updated knowledge on basic and advanced CPR, taking into account that the guidelines published by the AHA are modified based on scientific research conducted periodically and allow us to provide high quality CPR. Even so, training in the prevention of cardiorespiratory arrest (CPR) and basic CPR maneuvers in resident physicians is poorly developed (10).

The Sacred Heart of Jesus Hospital is a "basic hospital that provides clinical-surgical care and has outpatient, emergency, clinical and surgical hospitalization services; it has basic specialties (internal medicine, pediatrics, gynecology-obstetrics, general surgery, anesthesiology, clinical laboratory and imaging". It has 40 health professionals. Being a referral facility, it provides care to patients with different pathologies that are referred from centers of lower complexity; often adverse situations such as cardiorespiratory arrest occur and an immediate and timely response from professionals is necessary.

"Several articles have dealt with the problem worldwide. Studies have been carried out in England, the United States of America, Japan, New Zealand, Sweden and China, and have reached the same conclusion: there is a lack of training in CPR in undergraduate medical education programs, recently graduated physicians do not feel comfortable with resuscitation and make serious errors" (10).

Deaths from cardiopulmonary arrest for the year 2014 in the U.S. was 353,427 people (American Heart Association 2017). Not counting data from Ecuador. Because of these high values, there have been meetings and associations such as the AHA (American Heart Association) in order to analyze and provide treatment for cardiorespiratory arrest, through clear and timely protocols.

According to the 2017 AHA report and statistics about heart disease and stroke, including cardiac arrest on an annual average the cost was$199.6 billion (American Heart Association 2017), (18).

Lack of CPR knowledge plays an important role in the survival of the (Ramachandran et al. 2013). Therefore, knowledge about cardiopulmonary resuscitation is essential to perform quality resuscitation and avoid complications.

1.4. OBJECTIVES

1.4.1. GENERAL OBJECTIVE:

To determine the knowledge of basic and advanced cardiopulmonary resuscitation management in the health personnel of the emergency area in the Hospital Sagrado Corazón de Jesús Quevedo, in the period from August-September 2020.

1.4.2. SPECIFIC OBJECTIVES

- To evaluate the level of knowledge of health professionals in basic and advanced CPR management.

- To identify the shortcomings of health personnel in basic and advanced cardiopulmonary resuscitation.

- To estimate the relationship between the level of CPR knowledge and the length of work experience.

1.5.. HYPOTHESIS

Adult CPR training significantly influences the knowledge of emergency health care workers.

Training in cardiopulmonary resuscitation does not significantly influence the knowledge of emergency health workers.

Years of work experience influence the level of CPR knowledge.

Years of work experience do not influence the level of CPR knowledge.

The highest percentage of health professionals in the emergency area have a low level of knowledge of cardiopulmonary resuscitation.

The highest percentage of health professionals did not receive CPR training.

CHAPTER II

2. THEORETICAL FRAMEWORK

NATIONAL BACKGROUND

Dr. Cynthia Cabrera Jurado, Dr. Christopher Cedillo Carrión conducted a research study entitled: "level of knowledge on basic and advanced adult life support in members of surgical teams practicing in referral hospitals in the city of Quito in 2019" whose objective was "to determine the level of knowledge on basic and advanced adult life support in members of surgical teams practicing in referral hospitals in the city of Quito" in the months of February-March 2019. The type of study was multicenter, cross-sectional analytical. The population consisted of 126 professionals. The collection technique was the interview and the instrument used was a questionnaire. The conclusions were: they observed that about 79% among doctors and nurses know the importance of immediate and timely response protocol, 21% have no knowledge, from which they concluded that the knowledge in BLS can be said to be in a percentage where doctors and graduates of the hospital are in an acceptable average but not excellent for cardiorespiratory arrest care. (12)

INTERNATIONAL BACKGROUND:

María Dolores Lazo Caparrós, conducted a qualification study entitled "Level of knowledge and skills of cardiopulmonary resuscitation in workers", Spain 2017 in the month of September, whose objective was to obtain information on knowledge, skills and attitudes in the event that they encounter a person in CPR. The type of study was observational cross-sectional, the population consisted of a population 98 people, Staff working in the facilities of the Central Térmica Litoral Almería. Who have agreed to participate voluntarily in the study, the data collection technique was the interview and the instrument used were the surveys, the conclusions were that the comparison with the study of the Spanish council of cardiopulmonary resuscitation slightly more than half of the Spanish population over 18 years, specifically 55%, claims to know what is sudden cardiac arrest, compared to 44.8% who do not know. (María Dolores Lazo, 2017) (16)

German Aranzábal-Alegría, Araceli Verastegui-Díaz, Dante M. Quinones-Laveriano, Lizet Y. Quintana-Mendoza, Jennifer Vilchez-Cornejoc, Ciro B. Espejo, conducted a research study entitled: Factors associated with the level of knowledge in cardiopulmonary resuscitation in hospitals in Peru, Peru 2016, in the month of June, whose objective was to determine the association between

The type of study was a cross-sectional multicenter analytical cross-sectional study. The population was made up of health personnel from 25 hospitals in Peru. The study included health personnel who worked permanently in each hospital and who voluntarily agreed to participate. In addition, hospitals in 9 sites in the capital (Lima) and 13 sites in the provinces (Piura, La Libertad, Ucayali, Cusco) were included. Those who filled out the questionnaire incompletely or did not answer the CPR knowledge questions were excluded (25 surveys), the data collection technique was the interview and the instrument used was the surveys, the conclusions were that 59.0% (634) had a poor knowledge of CPR. The nurses had the highest scores (63%), followed by physicians (51%), medical interns (35%) and resident physicians (33%). (German Aranzábal-Alegría, Araceli Verastegui- Díaz, Peru 2016) (5).

Aldo López-González, Walter Delgado, conducted a research study entitled: Knowledge about basic and advanced adult cardiopulmonary resuscitation of resident physicians of a third level hospital, Paraguay 2017, whose objective was to determine the level of knowledge that resident physicians of the National Hospital of Itauguá have about basic and advanced cardiopulmonary resuscitation in adults, the type of study was observational, descriptive, cross-sectional, The population consisted of medical residents of the National Hospital of Itauguá, from different specialties, the data collection technique was the interview and the instrument used were surveys, the conclusions were that the medical residents of the National Hospital of Itauguá, participants of this study, found a very high unsatisfactory percentage (over 80%) of knowledge about cardiopulmonary resuscitation.(Aldo López-González, Walter Delgado, Paraguay 2017) (19) (19)

Balcázar, conducted a research study entitled: knowledge on basic and advanced cardiopulmonary resuscitation in health personnel, Mexico 2017, whose objective was to determine the level of knowledge of professional health personnel on cardiopulmonary resuscitation in the emergency service, the type of study was applicative, quantitative and descriptive, the population consisted of doctors and nursing graduates, the data collection technique was the interview and the instrument used were surveys, the conclusions were that 89.34% of the study population of health personnel demonstrated an unsatisfactory level of knowledge, thus exposing that there are very serious deficiencies in the knowledge of cardiopulmonary resuscitation, and that the years of experience and the ability in resuscitation are not associated with the level of knowledge. (Balcazar, American Heart Association, 2017). (17)

Dr. Idoris Cordero Escobar, "Several articles have addressed the problem worldwide. Studies have been conducted in England, United States of America, Japan, New Zealand, Sweden and China, the objective of this talk is to make an update on the teaching of cardiopulmonary and cerebral resuscitation, only theoretical knowledge of 41 doctors and 30 interns of sixth year of medicine was evaluated, a multiple choice test was used and it was only approved by 39% of the doctors and 10% of the interns. And they have reached the same conclusion: there is a lack of CPR training in undergraduate medical education programs, recently graduated physicians are not comfortable with resuscitation and make serious mistakes" (Dr.C. Idoris Cordero Escobar 2017). (10)

Carmen Escriba Mendoza, Wilbert Sulca Barrón, conducted a research study entitled: knowledge and skills in the management of basic CPR in nursing professionals in the health center Licenciados. Ayacucho. 2017, Peru 2017, whose objective was to determine the relationship between knowledge and skills in the management of Basic CPR in nursing professionals in the Centro De Salud Licenciados, Ayacucho, 2017. The type of study was Quantitative-Applied, the population consisted of 18 nursing professionals working in the emergency services of the Licenciados Health Center, Ayacucho, 2017, the data collection technique was the interview and the instrument used were the surveys ,the conclusions were ¨ The highest percentage of nursing professionals representing 61.Applying the chi2 test, it is demonstrated that there is no relationship between the level of knowledge with those who correctly and incorrectly perform basic CPR (P>0.05), rejecting the scientific hypothesis and accepting the null hypothesis ¨ (Carmen Escriba Mendoza, 2017) (20).

2.1. CARDIOPULMONARY RESUSCITATION

Cardiopulmonary resuscitation is defined as a sequential and organized response to cardiac arrest, of which will include:

- recognizing the absence of circulation and breathing

- basic life support with chest compressions and ventilations

- advanced cardiac life support in which there is definitive airway and rhythm control.

- treatment after resuscitation

Immediate initiation of uninterrupted continuous chest compressions and early defibrillation are paramount to success. The speed, efficiency, and correct application of CPR with minute interruptions will result in successful outcomes. (8)

2.2. CARDIORESPIRATORY ARREST

This will include any clinical situation in which there is an unexpected, abrupt and potentially reversible cessation of respiratory and cardiac functions in a spontaneous manner.

This arrest will not be the result of a natural evolution due to an advanced chronic pathology or one that is not curable, or on the other hand due to the aging of a person, and if it is not neutralized with resuscitation measures, this arrest will produce an abrupt reduction of oxygen transport that will lead to a hypoxia of the brain initially and then will lead to cellular lesions in the person's organism, due to tissue anoxia and biological death. (21)

2.3. PATHOPHYSIOLOGY OF PCR

Cardiorespiratory arrest is the interruption of the mechanical activity of the heart, which produces a decrease in the transport of oxygen to the cell primarily at the cerebral and cardiac level. This will cause the change of aerobic and anaerobic metabolism, with the congruent lower production of ATP molecules (adenosine triphosphate).

In the first 5 minutes after cardiac arrest the cellular ATP reserves have weakened. A small amount of energy will be obtained via AMP (adenosine monophosphate), which is converted to adenosine, which has lethal effects, depressing conduction through the atrioventricular node and causing arteriolar vasodilatation. The ATP-dependent ionic pumps will be lost, causing intracellular depletion of magnesium and potassium, inactivation of sodium channels and activation of calcium channels.

At myocardial height, we observe that coronary perfusion pressure is the best hemodynamic predictor of return to spontaneous circulation. With external cardiac massage it will reach about 5 to 10% of basal myocardial flow, rising to about 40% of the prepared condition with the use of vasopressor drugs such as (adrenaline). (22)

2.4. ETHIOPATHOLOGY

Cardiological	• acute myocardial infarction
	• arrhythmias (VF/VSVT, bradycardias, A-V block II and III degree) • pulmonary thrombo embolism • cardiac tamponade
Metabolic	• hypokalemia • hypercalcemia
Respiratory	• airway obstruction • depressionfrom respiratory center • bronchoaspiration • choking or suffocation • tension pneumothorax • respiratory insufficiency
Traumatic	• cranioencephalic • thoracic • great vessel injury • internal or external bleeding
Shcok **Hypothermia** **Iatrogenic**	• overdosage of anesthetic agents

Cardiorespiratory arrest or cardiac arrest (CRA) is characterized as a clinical situation in which there is an abrupt, reversible and unexpected interruption of the mechanical activity of the heart and spontaneous breathing. (23)

2.4.1.　　　BASIC PEDIATRIC CARDIO PULMONARY RESUSCITATION

In pediatric patients, cardiac arrest is usually the consequence of impaired respiratory and circulatory functions that will be secondary to a pathology or an accident.

In order to reduce the morbimortality of CA in paediatrics, we will use the chain of survival, thus applying preventive measures, anticipation, providing basic life support and CPR techniques. Thus activating emergency teams and establishing advanced life support measures that include airway control, early defibrillation, oxygenation, drugs and fluids as soon as possible. (24)

BASIC LIFE SUPPORT

This is characterized by a set of techniques that allow to recognize and act on a CPR without specific equipment until the arrival of qualified health personnel. A correct application of CPR will reduce morbidity and mortality.

2.4.2.   EPIDEMIOLOGY

Cardiorespiratory arrest in children is unusual. The incidence of out-of-hospital cardiorespiratory arrest is considered to be 8-20 cases per 100,000 children. (25)

2.4.3.   WHAT ARE THE CAUSES

There are a number of circumstances that will cause a child's heartbeat and breathing to stop. Situations where we may need to perform CPR on a child include:(26)

- In the case of asphyxiation
- Electric shock
- Drowning
- Head Trauma
- Excessive bleeding
- Lung disease
- Hot flush
- Intoxication

2.4.4.   SYMPTOMS

Cardiopulmonary resuscitation should be performed if the child has any of these symptoms :(26)

- Respiratory arrest
- Cognitive loss
- No pulse

PRIMARY EVALUATION

This assessment uses the following abbreviations ABCDE

- By air
- Breathing
- Circulation

- Disability (neurological status)
- Exhibition

THE AIRWAY

For the assessment of the airway is essential to decide whether it is patent, sustainable or non-sustainable.

- Patent: is patent when the airway is completely clear with normal breathing.
- Sustainable: it is sustainable when the airway can be preserved with simple patency maneuvers.
- Non-sustainable: it is not sustainable when the airway requires advanced maneuvers for its management. (27)

BREATHING

For the assessment of breathing you will understand:

- Respiratory rate
- Breathing effort
- Tidal volume
- Airway and lung sounds
- Pulse Oximetry

CIRCULATION

For the assessment of circulation will comprise cardiovascular function and organ perfusion.

To assess cardiovascular function we must observe the following parameters:

- Skin coloration and temperature
- Capillary filling
- Peripheral and central pulse quality
- Blood pressure

DISABILITY (NEUROLOGICAL CONDITION)

The neurological status will include the assessment of 2 components of the central nervous system: the cortex and the brain stem.

For this valuation will include:

1. AVDI
- Alert
- Respond to the voice
- Responding to pain
- Unconsciousness
2. The Glasgow Coma Scale
3. Pupillary response to light

EXHIBITION

Remove the child's clothing for exposure. Assess the child from head to toe and observe the front and back. Once fully assessed, the child should be covered to avoid hypothermia.

The appearance of bleeding, indirect signs of abuse, burns should be assessed, always bearing in mind the mobilization of polytraumatized patients or any risk of cervical trauma. (27)

HOW SHOULD WE ACT?

In that case the first thing to do is to confirm the patient's state of consciousness, we will speak loudly very close to the ears or we will stimulate the patient in a gentle way.

But if we suspect the presence of a cervical injury, we must perform a bimanual immobilization before stimulating the patient. If the patient responds, we will leave him/her in a safe position, reporting what has happened and activating emergency equipment. If the patient does not respond, we will perform the following maneuvers:

- We place the patient in the supine position on a flat, hard, smooth surface.
- We open the airway by means of the forehead - chin maneuver and place one hand on the forehead and gently tilt the head back, making an extension of the neck, it is done moderately in children and neutral in infants.
- Immediately raise the chin with the tips of the index and middle fingers of the other hand (in case of trauma, raise the angles of the jaw upwards and forwards, best with two fingers of each hand, while fixing the neck).
- If the presence of a foreign body is evident, it will only be removed if it is visible and can be easily extracted, thus avoiding blind sweeping.
- Keeping the patient with the airways open we will approach the mouth and nose to check for normal breathing, no more than 10 seconds.
- Then we should look to see if the child raises the chest and abdomen.
- We will listen for the presence of breath sounds.
- Let's feel the exhaled air on our cheek.

If the child is breathing normally, we will place him/her in a lateral safety position which will prevent the tongue from falling out.

We will also avoid any pressure on the thorax and extremities, then after about 30 minutes we will change sides. If it is traumatic we will leave him in the position he is in and in a safe way, we will activate the emergency equipment and we will monitor the child's breathing frequently. (24)

- If there is no normal breathing, we will perform ventilations, either with exhaled air or instrumental airway support and oxygen therapy. Ventilations with exhaled air (FIO2 60rpm), we will perform exclusively ventilations (12 -20/min) continuously revaluating.
- If there are no signs of life or pulse less than 60 bpm, we will start chest compressions combined with ventilations (15/2).

<u>CHEST COMPRESSIONS</u>

Chest compressions will be performed on the lower half of the sternum, placing both thumbs above the xiphoid processes, hugging the thorax with both hands, thus adapting to the size and age.

That pressure that is exerted should depress the sternum by at least one third of the anteroposterior diameter of the thorax (approximately 4 cm in infants, 5 cm in children and up to 6 cm in adults), the rhythm that will be carried out will be of
100 to 120 bpm, thus using the same pressure time as decompression time.

It is very important to emphasize that the usefulness of mechanical compression or depth measurement devices is more controversial in pediatrics:

IN INFANTS

In infants, we will perform chest compressions with two fingers perpendicular to the thorax, or by holding the thorax with two hands supporting both thumbs.

IN CHILDREN

In children we will place the heel of one hand on the compression area and we will keep the arm extended vertically to the chest, if necessary we will use both hands, thus placing the heel of one hand on the other without leaning on it, thus avoiding injury to the ribs. (24)

- In this way we will combine compressions with 15/2 ventilations in infants and children, or 30/2 in adults.

- Every two minutes we will confirm the effectiveness of CPR using no more than 10 seconds.

2.4.5.　　　PRONOSTICO

Unfavourably the survival of a child who has suffered a cardiopulmonary arrest is greatly reduced to only approximately 25% in in-hospital CRA and 10% in out-of-hospital CRA. The components that will contribute if a child overcomes a cardiorespiratory arrest include:

- Anticipated clinical status of the child, if it was first healthy it has a better prognosis.
- Respiratory causes are better predicted than cardiac arrests.
- It is important to calculate the time that has elapsed until basic and advanced CPR maneuvers are initiated.
- The quality of resuscitation maneuvers and intensive post-resuscitation meticulousness. (25)

AUTOMATED EXTERNAL DEFIBRILLATION (AED)

Once the AED has arrived, turn it on and follow the instructions below:

- In children over 8 years old or weighing 25 kg we will apply DEA with adult patches.

- In children between 1 and 8 years of age we will use the available AED, preferably with attenuators or pediatric pads with a charge of (50 -75 Joules).

- In infants the use of AED is acceptable, but preferably with attenuated.

In this way we will minimize interruptions in chest compressions, thus following the indications of the AED and leave the patches on the chest until help arrives.

It is very important:

- Do not discontinue BLS with or without an AED until there are clear signs of life or a pulse greater than 60 beats per minute with effective breathing.

- Do not stop BLS with or without an AED until qualified equipment arrives that can take over the situation.

- Do not stop BLS with or without an AED until you are exhausted or unsafe.

- Do not stop BLS with or without an AED until there are clear biological signs of death.

2.5. PEDIATRIC ADVANCED CARDIO PULMONARY RESUSCITATION

The goal of advanced life support is the definitive treatment of cardiorespiratory arrest. It will only be applied by highly trained personnel and with the appropriate equipment until respiratory function and spontaneous circulation are restored.

Working safely and as a team, these techniques include high quality chest compressions, good maintenance of a patent airway and its definitive isolation, including oxygenation, ventilation, monitoring for diagnosis and treatment of arrhythmias, and vascular access to administer fluids and drugs. We can use ultrasound especially to detect cardiac activity and any other potentially treatable causes of cardiac arrest in no more than 10 seconds in a much more organized manner. (24)

PAEDIATRIC ADVANCED LIFE SUPPORT PROCESS OPTIMISATION OF

AIRWAY AND VENTILATION

We must perform the chin front maneuver or jaw traction, the use of oro-pharyngeal cannula and ventilation with a self-inflating bag, mask and 100% oxygen are the first techniques that are recommended for the control of both the airway and ventilation, and these must be maintained until definitive control.

The most effective and safest method of airway isolation, sustainability and control is intubation, and should be performed by highly experienced trainers. (28)

AIRWAY OPENING DEVICES

Oropharyngeal cannula: This cannula, when introduced into the oral cavity, will allow us to keep the airway open and ventilate with the mask. While performing the chin front maneuver we will choose the size (00-5), thus measuring the distance between the angle of the mandible and the height of the upper incisors.

- In infants it will be introduced with the convexity upwards and we will use a depressor or a laryngoscope blade.

- In children it will be introduced with the concavity upwards and in the soft palate we will rotate at 180 degrees until the correct position is obtained.

Nasopharyngeal Cannula: The use of this cannula is very infrequent, it is going to be measured from the nostrils to the tragus. It is very important to know that it should not be used in coagulopathies or fractures of the skull base.

Face Mask: These masks are usually transparent and are adapted to the age (they are round in infants and triangular in children), should allow a good seal to the face (inflatable base) and also a good grip area with the hand (one finger in the nasal area, the second finger in the buccal / mental area of the mask and the third, fourth and fifth finger should be placed in the mandibular area of the patient.

Oxygen therapy: the oxygen concentration for cardiopulmonary resuscitation ventilations will be 100% (flow 15L / min).

Aspiration of secretions or vomit: This aspiration will be preferable with flexible probes and a device, thus controlling the pressure (80-120mmHg) and under direct visualization. Rigid probes will be useful in vomiting or when there is food debris. (28)

Endotracheal Intubation:

In this case, the oro-tracheal route will do the most indicated and will certify an adequate ventilation and oxygen supply, and this will avoid gastric distension and pulmonary aspiration. No pre-medication will be needed.

- This intubation technique should be performed by highly experienced personnel, should not last more than 30 seconds and without chest compressions for no more than 10 seconds.

We are going to prepare the necessary material, we are going to calculate the size/internal calibre of the endotracheal tube with tape or ruler. We are going to prepare tubes of superior and inferior calibers and preferably with pneumotaping (except in neonates) since they propose greater advantages in children with low pulmonary distensibility or who have high resistance in the airway, or if they present air leaks in the glottis. All this will allow a smaller caliber error and a better monitoring.

Exaggerated pneumotap pressure may cause laryngeal tissue ischemia and secondary stenosis. It is for this reason that balloon inflation pressure (lower 25 with H_2O) should be monitored.

- We will place the patient in an aligned position with the head in moderate or neutral extension depending on their age.

- We will pre-oxygenate 100% with bag-mask ventilation.

- We will intubate and check the correct placement of the endotracheal tube.

- With the endotracheal tube, it will not be necessary for rescuers to synchronize the rhythm of compressions and ventilations as much (15/2). It will continue to quality chest compressions at 100-120 per minute and ventilations at 10 per minute independently.

- Once the position of the endotracheal tube is confirmed, we are going to fix it and we are going to recheck it, we are going to avoid both the flexion of the head (it introduces more the tube) and the extension (it displaces it outwards) then we are going to proceed to the aspiration of secretions.

- In case of suspicion of abnormal intubation or if auscultation is asymmetrical (hypoventilation on the left side), remove 0.5 cm by 0.5 cm and assess. In case of doubt, we remove the tube and ventilate with bag and mask.

• Nowadays the video laryngoscope can facilitate intubation.

• Rarely it will require surgical access to the airway.

• Emergency cricothyroidotomy will only be applied in the case of not being able to intubate due to an obstruction or foreign body in the glottis, facial trauma, etc.).

- It is important to emphasize that intubation may be indicated in other conditions that will require a safe airway (non-sustainable airway, in the case of mechanical ventilation needs, exhausted patients, hemodynamic decompensation, Glasgow less than 9, CO2 control, intracranial pressure.

- In this case we will use a rapid sequence of intubation, with Induction Pharmacology to coma, combining anesthetics, muscle relaxants, sedatives that will reduce the risk of failure.

2.5.1.   DRUGS, FLUIDS AND INFUSION ROUTE IN ADVANCED LIFE SUPPORT.

• In paediatric cardiopulmonary resuscitation, isotonic crystalloids are the recommended fluids, in boluses of 20 ml/kg.

• Adrenaline is still the drug of choice in CPR, and the dose is still maintained at 10 mg/kg (diluted and maximum 1 mg) every 3-5 min in all types of rhythms (it has been proven that higher doses will not improve survival or neurological prognosis).

• For defibrillable rhythms we will use amiodarone, which is administered in boluses of 5mg/kg (the first dose immediately after the third defibrillation and the fifth if appropriate, adrenaline should also be administered).

• The drug that remains as an alternative to amiodarone is lidocaine in doses of 1mg/kg, maximum 100 mg.

• Atropine will not be considered a drug for cardiopulmonary resuscitation and its use will be restricted to bradycardias or vagal block.

- As for the use of sodium bicarbonate, there is no evidence that its use improves CPR outcomes and its use should be avoided for routine use. (28)

CHECK MATERIALS

A protocol for periodic verification of material and medication should be implemented, specifically listing the responsible personnel and a checklist of material and their responses. It is essential to review the material and medication after each CPR.

No equipment on the crash cart should be used for anything other than CPR and life-saving emergencies.

PERSONNEL PREPARATION

All medical, nursing and auxiliary professionals should undergo periodic training and recycling, not only in paediatric and neonatal CPR techniques, but also in the distribution of material and medication in the crash cart and its use during CPR. (29)

2.6. CARDIOPULMONARY RESUSCITATION IN ADULTS

Basic life support is the set of actions, which includes knowledge of the response system to a medical emergency and knowledge of the initial actions to be taken in situations such as: State of persistent or recovered unconsciousness, severe trauma, respiratory arrest and cardiorespiratory arrest".

The characteristic of this is that it is carried out without any equipment, accepting only the use of accessories to prevent mouth-to-mouth or mouth-to-nose contact between the rescuer and the victim (barrier devices) or the use of the automatic defibrillator. (30).

In the study on basic CPR, published in the Revista Médica de Chile, only 41 physicians and 30 sixth year interns were evaluated for theoretical knowledge, a multiple choice test was used and only 39% of the physicians and 10% of the interns passed (31).

Another study, whose objective was to evaluate the level of theoretical knowledge and practical skills in CPR in a sample of residents in Spain, concluded that it seems necessary to establish more effective instructional methods, where the use of simulated clinical scenarios can be a useful tool to improve learning, such as the evaluation of the terminal competencies of the medical graduate (32).

2.6.2.   IN-HOSPITAL CARDIOPULMONARY RESUSCITATION OF THE ADULT PATIENT

CARDIAC ARREST PREVENTION AND RAPID RESPONSE SYSTEMS

It is important to recognize when clinical deterioration occurs, this is critical in the prevention of cardiac arrest in the in-hospital setting. Recognition and rapid response systems have been developed. The first system originated in Australia and then was created in different institutions in various countries.

According to the international committee, hospitals should have a rapid response system consisting of:

a. System that allows the recognition of clinical deterioration with criteria for all staff.

b. Mechanism for activation of rescue systems, available to health personnel and family members or acquaintances.

c. Response mechanism for correct management (33).

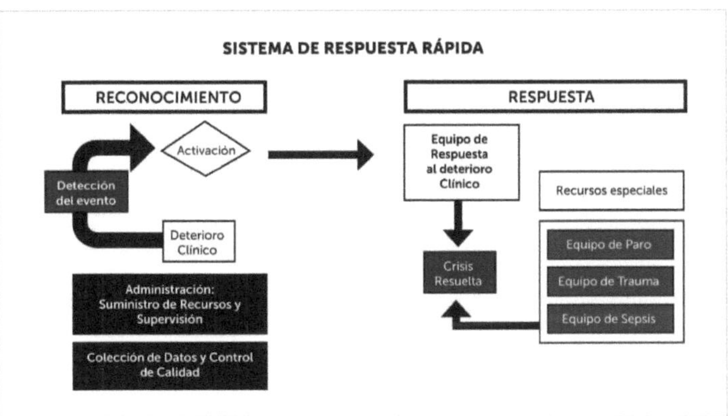

Illustration 1. Rapid Response Systems
Adapted from DeVita et al. Adapted from DeVita et al. Findings from the first consensus conference on emergency medical teams. Crit care med2006; 34:2463-78.

To recognize clinical deterioration, methods based on the alteration of physiological parameters are used, identifying predefined values accompanied by other manifestations such as use of accessory respiratory muscles, altered state of consciousness, decreased diuresis. These parameter alterations are reflected in the vital signs, which may be high or low values (for example, HR <8 or > 28 rpm, pulse oximetry <90%, SBP < 80 or > 200 mmHg, HR <40 or >140 bpm, among others (33).

There are other methods in which points are added based on the degree of alteration of physiological parameters and the trigger threshold depends on these. Most systems have rescue teams that assess and provide treatment at the patient's site. These teams are composed of respiratory therapists, nurses, internal medicine or intensive care fellows (residents), and mixed teams. Systems have been organized around the intensive care unit. When a patient's clinical deterioration occurs in any area within the hospital, a call is made to the center that immediately triggers the activation of the rapid response system. This call is transferred to the ICU (intensive care unit), the nurse is in charge of assessing the reason for the call and the patient's condition, the resident physician together with the attending physician will examine the patient and decide on the procedure to be followed. Many patients require care in a more complex unit (33).

CPR MANOEUVRES AND THEIR CLINICAL APPLICATION

the likelihood of restoring cardiac function and achieving survival with adequate neurological function, regardless of the cause of cardiac arrest, depends primarily on the speed with which the event is recognized and quality cardiopulmonary resuscitation maneuvers are initiated, as well as post-arrest management once circulation has been restored (32).

2.6.3.   HOW TO RECOGNIZE CARDIAC ARREST:

It must be fast and simple, it is based on the absence of the response to tactile and verbal stimuli (31), also a breathing that is not normal is frequently presented, agonal breathing is developed, this is developed by cerebral hypoxia and reflects the liberation of several nervous centers that are normally suppressed, it is given by the simultaneous and intense activation of the inspiratory muscles. The agonal breathing generates a beneficial effect through ventilation and blood flow that produces, achieving the success of resuscitation maneuvers. The low sensitivity and specificity of pulse detection is a point of contention and is not recommended. Medical personnel and the professional rescuer should be taught, but the rescuer should not take more than 10 seconds or they may skip it and begin resuscitation. Performing chest compressions on people who are not in cardiac arrest may cause slight damage to the rib cage, so it is advisable to initiate resuscitation when in doubt (34).

SIGNS AND SYMPTOMS:
Most victims of CRA usually have no symptoms, sometimes just before the event. Symptoms include sudden loss of consciousness, absent pulse, and no breathing. Some symptoms usually occur within an hour before CRA: tachycardia, dizziness, dyspnea, nausea or vomiting, chest pain. (35)

BASIC CPR

The chain of survival has the vital links that are necessary for successful resuscitation. These links are mostly applied in cases of patients with primary cardiac arrest and asphyxia, they are 4 links in the following order:

1.   Early recognition and calling for help: we must know how to recognize when it is a chest pain of cardiac origin and immediately call emergency just before the patient collapses, to arrive as soon as possible and prevent CRA from occurring at that time, and achieve a high survival rate.

2.   Early control CPR: Initiating CPR maneuvers doubles patient survival after CPR. If trained, the bystander should initiate chest compressions along with ventilations.

3.   Early defibrillation: If defibrillation is performed within the first 3 to 5 minutes of collapse, the chance of survival is high, 50 to 70%. It can be accomplished with a public access AED (automated external defibrillator).

4.   Early ALS (Advanced Life Support) and post-resuscitation care or management: when BLS is unsuccessful, it is necessary to proceed to ALS where airway management, drug administration and correction of causal factors are performed (30).

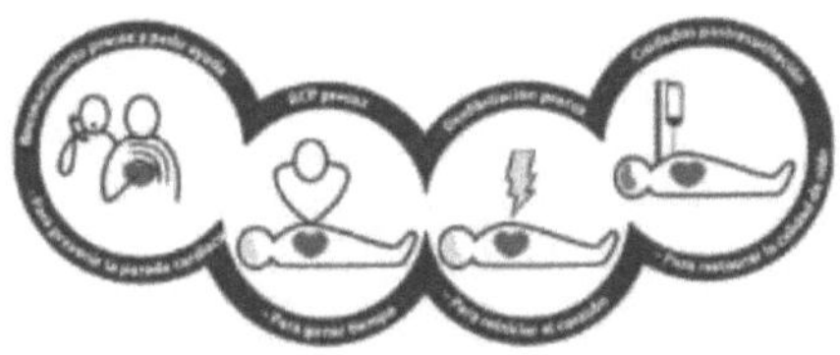

Illustration 2. Chain of survival taken from: Guidelines for resuscitation 2015

The main characteristic is that it is performed without any equipment, only the use of barrier devices that prevent mouth-to-mouth or mouth-to-nose contact between the victim and the resuscitator or the use of the automatic defibrillator is accepted (30).

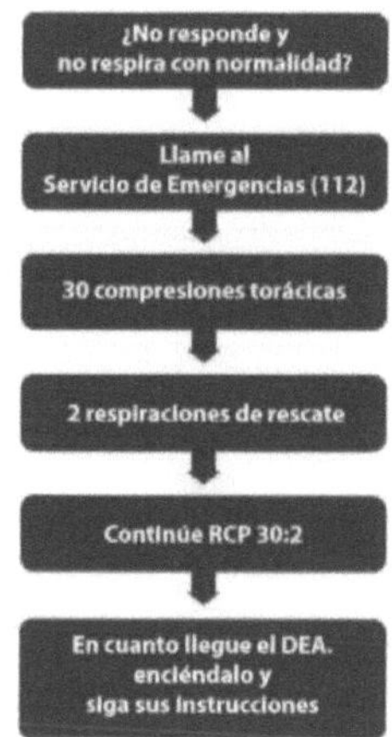

Ilustración 2 . Algoritmo de Soporte vital básico, tomado de: Guidelines for resuscitation 2015

Illustration 3. Basic life support algorithm, taken from: Guidelines for resuscitation 2015

In this case, the most important thing to do is to check if the victim is unresponsive, not breathing or has abnormal breathing or simply whimpers. If more than one rescuer is present, the first rescuer should check for the presence of a pulse during the first 10 seconds and if not present should begin chest compressions and ventilations in a 30:2 ratio. The second rescuer will be in charge of activating the emergency response system (EMS) and obtaining an AED; if a third rescuer is available, he or she will open the airway and provide the 2 ventilations. If a pulse is present but breathing is absent, the airway should be opened and rescue ventilation provided every 5 to 6 seconds in adults. (35)

• **Checking breathing and opening the airway:** Quickly check that the person who collapsed responds to the call or stimulus and if they are breathing normally or abnormally. Using the chin-forehead maneuver or jaw thrust, open the airway to check if the person is breathing or if there is the presence of a foreign object. (30) If there is a suspicion of cervical injury, "The mandibular traction maneuver is a technique to open the airway by placing the fingers behind the mandibular angle and lifting the mandible. "(35).

• **Chest compressions are started:** After CPR there is a cessation of blood flow and blood remains in the lungs, on the other hand, it remains oxygenated blood that is in the arterial system for a few minutes. Cardiac compressions keep the oxygenated blood circulating while breathing and cardiac fusion are restored. (35) For this reason it is important to start chest compressions before ventilations. The following are the steps for performing manual chest compressions:

1. Compressions are done in the center of the chest.
2. Compressions are made to a depth of 2 inches (5 cm), not to exceed 2 inches (6 cm).
3. It compresses at a rate of 100-120 compressions per minute, avoiding interruptions.
4. The thorax must be allowed to re-expand completely after compression; do not rest on the thorax during re-expansion (30). Hand position: In the adult, the "heel of the hand in the center of the chest with the other hand on top" is placed on the lower half of the sternum. If there is only one rescuer, he/she should kneel next to the patient, thus favoring compressions and ventilations, as well as avoiding interruptions. (30)

Ventilation: There are two situations: if the patient achieves effective breathing, he/she is placed in the lateral safety position and if he/she is not breathing, 2 ventilations should be administered to raise the thorax, separated allowing the victim to exhale between each ventilation. After the 2 ventilations, quickly continue with chest compression. (35)

Face Mask: Although the risk of infection from CPR is low, the health care team must take all standard precautions to avoid exposure to body fluids such as blood. Therefore, it is important to use a facemask or bag-mask system for delivery of ventilations. Training is required to use these devices; the ventilation rate is 1 breath per second, a total of 10 breaths per minute).

Early defibrillation: AED (automated external defibrillator) defibrillation is part of comprehensive BLS care (21). It is performed on the unconscious CRA victim. It is indicated in the two types of defibrillable CRA rhythms which are: fibrillation or pulseless ventricular tachycardia, which if not treated in time are fatal.

Defibrillator according to the access route:

- **External** defibrillator-Energy is delivered through paddles or electrodes that are placed on the skin surface of the chest.
- **Automatic external defibrillator:** This may be semi-automatic, capable of detecting the arrhythmia and informing the operator and releasing energy, or it may be fully automatic and require no operator intervention in the release of energy. (35)

Defibrillator according to the type of energy:

- **Two-phase:** Just before reversing an energy current is discharged in the positive direction, then in the remaining milliseconds a negative energy current flows. They are more efficient than single-phase as they require half the energy. If the dose is unknown, use 200 joules. In children, 2 to 4 Joules / Kg will be applied in the case of defibrillation and 0.5 to 1 J / Kg in cardioversion.

- **Single-phase:** These are the most commonly used, they discharge energy current in one direction (unipolar). The dose used is 360 joules.

Defibrillable rhythms:

• **Ventricular fibrillation:** The heart has a disorganized electrical activity, where the myocardial cells contract in a disorderly manner and is represented as irregular waves on the ECG (electrocardiogram).
• **Pulseless ventricular tachycardia:** Electrical activity occurs in the heart that causes the myocardial cells to contract, which is not enough to perform their pump function. The ECG shows wide, high-frequency QRS waves of 200 per minute or more.

These two types of tachyarrhythmias are the most frequent in out-of-hospital cardiac arrest and where the effective treatment is defibrillation and is a function of time. Survival and success is between 49-75%. In the out-of-hospital setting defibrillation should be performed within 5 minutes of the onset of the event and in the in-hospital setting within 3 minutes. With each minute of delay in defibrillation, the survival rate to discharge decreases by 10-15%. Therefore, it is important that public places with a large number of people have an AED.

Contraindications to defibrillation:

- CRA with asystole, in this case there is no electrical activity and no blood pumping. A flat isoelectric line is visualized on the ECG.
- Pulseless Electrical Activity (PEA) is any electrical activity, but no blood pumping. (45)

The frequency of in-hospital cardiac arrest caused by pulseless ventricular fibrillation or tachycardia is lower than that of out-of-hospital, and occurs in 25%, in terms of prognosis is higher compared to cardiac arrest with organized pulseless electrical activity or asystole. For this reason it is important to have the ability to quickly recognize and administer a non-synchronized electric shock in these patients, considered a priority intervention that should be performed even before the rescue team arrives. Automatic external defibrillators are considered an alternative to manual defibrillators and can be used by untrained personnel, basic cardiopulmonary resuscitation maneuvers should be initiated quickly while the defibrillator is deployed. (36)

2.6.4.   BASIC RESUSCITATION MANEUVERS:

When blood flow ceases as a result of cardiac arrest, tissue ischemia occurs, which is greater in the heart and brain, as these are the most affected.

require a greater demand for energy. Time plays a very important role, as the delay in performing BLS decreases survival and if the victim survives, the neurological state will be altered. For this reason, it is important to activate the intrahospital rescue system once cardiac arrest has been recognized and basic CPR (cardiopulmonary resuscitation) maneuvers are initiated while the rescue team arrives. The objective of BLS is to maintain blood flow through chest compression maneuvers and ensure perfusion of target organs such as the heart and brain, increasing the victim's survival and reducing neurological sequelae (33).

To perform chest compressions the patient must be on a flat and firm surface, these are done at a depth of 5 and 6 cm, with a frequency of 100 and 120 per minute, in this way the thorax re-expansion is achieved and interruptions are reduced, the percentage of time that the compressions are done should not be less than 60% (34).

When the cause is primary and this occurs suddenly and witnessed, there is a reserve of oxygen in the blood, lungs and tissues at the time of circulatory cessation. Thanks to gas mobilization through agonal respirations and chest compressions, this oxygen reserve is renewed while the airway remains open. It is this oxygen reserve that allows resuscitation with chest compressions alone while the rescue team arrives. Based on preclinical studies, the oxygen reserve is likely to last 4 to 6 minutes. Individuals are trained in rescue ventilation, which should be performed in conjunction with chest compressions (34). The ratio of chest compressions to ventilations is 30 compressions followed by 2 ventilations in patients without an established airway. In the in-hospital setting there are several mechanisms of cardiac arrest (Table 1) mainly due to extracardiac causes (37), it is reasonable to use rescue ventilation during in-hospital CPR, but according to a recent cohort study in more than 10,000 patients showed a negative effect associated with attempted tracheal intubation during the first 15 minutes of in-hospital CPR (38), it is possible that it is related to interruptions during resuscitation in intubation attempts.

TABLE 1. CARDIAC AND NON-CARDIAC CAUSES OF PCR.

CAUSAS CARDIACAS	CAUSAS NO CARDIACAS
Enfermedad coronaria	Paro respiratorio.
Infarto del miocardio	Depresión respiratoria por drogas
Shock cardiogénico	Cuerpo extraño en vía aérea
Fibrilación ventricular	Epiglotitis.
Aneurisma disecante de la aorta	Quemaduras vías respiratorias
Endocarditis subaguda	Inhalación de tóxicos (CO)
ICC Refractaria	Inmersión
Taponamiento cardíaco	Embolia pulmonar
Ruptura ventricular o del séptum IV	Traumatismos de cráneo
Tumores cardíacos	Accidente Cerebro Vascular.(ACV)
Bloqueos auriculoventriculares	Epilepsia (status convulsivo)
Actividad eléctrica sin pulso	Hipoglicemia, Hipoxia
Taquicardia ventricular	Shock séptico fulminante
Taquiarritmias supraventriculares	Hipercalcemia
Asistolia	Shock eléctrico

Table 1. Cardiac and non-cardiac causes obtained from the adult basic cardiopulmonary resuscitation manual (2009) Padre Hurtado Hospital.

2.7. ADVANCED CPR

It is a set of therapeutic measures aimed at the treatment of cardiorespiratory arrest. It requires specific equipment and training. Quality CPR in adults increases the survival of the victim of arrest by means of 2 actions: basic life support and early defibrillation in pulseless ventricular fibrillation and tachycardia. Drug administration and advanced airway management have not been shown to increase survival, but should be included in training (30).

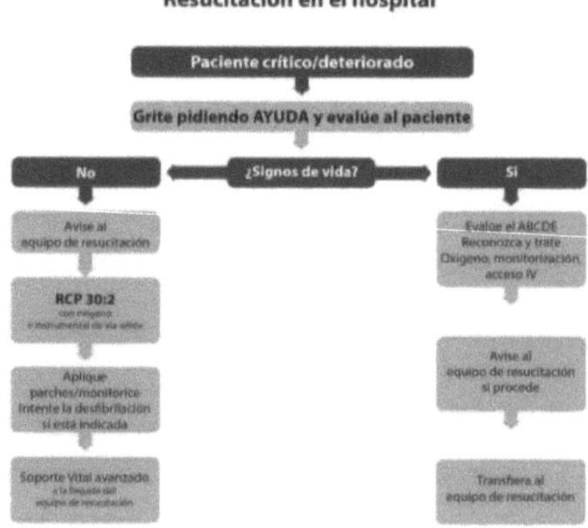

Ilustración 3. Algoritmo de resucitación hospitalaria tomado de: Guidelines for resuscitation 2015

Hospital resuscitation algorithm taken from: Guidelines for resuscitation 2015

2.7.1 PATHOPHYSIOLOGICAL ASPECTS OF ADVANCED CPR:

The amount of blood flow generated by chest compression maneuvers is limited, rarely exceeding 25% of cardiac output (CO), which does not meet metabolic demands. When circulation ceases immediately, the intense neuro-humoral response is triggered, which activates the adrenergic system and the release of vasopressin that produces a redistribution of blood flow to the heart and brain which are vital organs, this is achieved through vasoconstriction of non-vital territories such as skeletal muscle, splanchnic territory and skin (33).

Vasoconstrictors are required in most resuscitations, but despite these efforts, myocardial ischemia persists in resuscitation, may be attenuated if coronary flow is increased, but is only reversed when spontaneous circulation and coronary flow are reestablished. Adrenaline is currently the recommended vasoconstrictor, as evidence based on scientific information has not demonstrated a superior benefit to vasopressin. Adrenaline has a vasoconstrictor effect mediated by α1- and α2-adrenergic receptors, it also activates β1- and β2-adrenergic receptors. In the myocardium, β1-adrenergic receptors are found, which are responsible for stimulating contractile function (38). According to recent preclinical and clinical studies it has been demonstrated that adrenaline allows the restoration of cardiac activity, but post-cardiac arrest myocardial function will be compromised, therefore, the patient's survival. Unlike vasopressin it does not activate adrenergic receptors, but it has a long half-life, therefore, the vasoconstrictor effect will persist in the post-resuscitation period and an increase in afterload is generated compromising ventricular function. Even with the disadvantages, vasoconstrictors are used in CPR (33).

During resuscitation, blood flow is low and also decreases over time, for various reasons, such as loss of rib cage elasticity, which in turn compromises venous return, and loss of myocardial distensibility that compromises preload, so that chest compressions are not sufficient to maintain blood flow. But there is a window of time in which it is possible to restore the heart's activity through conventional resuscitation maneuvers. When the rescuers do not perform quality maneuvers, this complicates the problem even more (39). Mechanical devices have been invented to achieve quality resuscitation, and these have advantages over manual CPR, which often involves fatigue and inconsistency on the part of rescuers. In addition, during the transfer of the patient in cardiac arrest in motion allows us to perform invasive interventions (40).

Extracorporeal circulation makes it possible to provide normal blood flow levels and thus easily restore cardiac activity even when conventional resuscitation has failed, according to recent studies.

It has been demonstrated that extracorporeal circulation achieves high survival in cases refractory to conventional CPR maneuvers (41), but its use is limited due to cost. Extracorporeal circulation stabilizes the patient in cardiac arrest and allows diagnostic and therapeutic procedures to be performed during CPR (41).

MONITORING DURING CPR

Through physiological monitoring it is possible to optimize the effectiveness of cardiopulmonary resuscitation by adjusting the technique and deciding whether specific interventions are necessary (33).

"CAPNOGRAPHY AND MEASUREMENT OF FINAL EXHALED CO2:

It is the measurement of the partial pressure of CO_2 in the airway during the respiratory cycle and its graphical representation. The final exhaled CO_2 corresponds to the alveolar gas, provided that expiration is not interrupted by the next inspiration as in the case of patients with airway disease and gas trapping. The final exhaled CO_2 is determined by the following factors: CO_2 production at the tissue level which depends on metabolic activity, CO_2 transport from the tissues to the lungs which depends on blood flow, the percentage of alveolar dead space and pulmonary ventilation" (33).

During resuscitation, CO_2 production and dead space remain constant; therefore, the amount of final exhaled CO_2 will depend on the blood flow generated and the ventilation provided. In this way, the final exhaled CO_2 allows us to estimate the blood flow generated and if it is necessary to optimize CPR maneuvers, for example, when inadequate chest compressions are being performed, incomplete thoracic re-expansion or some mechanism that blocks blood flow (42).

Several studies show that a lower end-expiratory CO_2 value <10 mmHg predicts failure of resuscitation maneuvers and maneuvers should be optimized to achieve an increase in end-expiratory CO_2 value above 20 mmHg (Table 2) (43).

TABLE 2. CARDIOPULMONARY RESUSCITATION QUALITY MATRIX

Direct arterial pressure during thoracic decompression phase	>25mmHg
Final exhaled CO_2	>20mmHg
PARAMETER	VALUE
Continuity of chest compression	Compression fraction >60%.
Frequency of chest compression	100 to 120 compressions per minute
Depth of chest compression	5 to 6 cm
Thoracic Re-expansion	Completely avoid leaning on the thorax.

TABLE 2. Taken from Meany et al.
Quality of cardiopulmonary resuscitation: improving outcomes of cardiac resuscitation both in and out of the hospital: an American Heart Association consensus statement. Circulation.

It must be taken into account that when adrenaline is administered, the final exhaled CO2 will decrease little by little, due to an increase in afterload that decreases blood flow and also produces an increase in the alveolar dead space (44). On the other hand, when sodium bicarbonate is administered, the final exhaled CO2 increases due to a reaction with the protons present in the circulation which produce CO2. (45).

Capnography allows verification of correct placement of the endotracheal tube; it is the most recommended method, since it has a sensitivity and specificity close to 100%. It is also used in the verification of airway patency in ventilation with mask and auto-inflatable bag (33).

DIRECT BLOOD PRESSURE

Resuscitation maneuvers can be guided by BP (blood pressure) when the arresting patient is monitored in the in-hospital setting or those who have an arterial catheter placed during resuscitation. Chest compressions generate a coronary flow that depends on the coronary perfusion pressure, given by the gradient between aortic pressure and right atrial pressure in the thoracic decompression phase. The arterial pressure in the decompression phase will depend on the amount of blood ejected from the previous compression and the peripheral vascular resistance, so it is very important to perform chest compressions and the use of vasoconstrictor agents correctly. According to preclinical and clinical studies it has been demonstrated that there is a threshold of coronary perfusion pressure of 15 mmHg, with which it is impossible to restore cardiac activity. If direct measurement of right atrial pressure is not available, a value of 10 mmHg can be left and CPR maneuvers can be directed to achieve a BP during decompression with a level >25 mmHg (46).

With direct BP monitoring, it is preferable to administer a vasoconstrictor agent to exceed this critical threshold level of 25 mmHg (Table 2), but this invasive BP monitoring with adrenaline administration has only been done in animals (47). Thanks to the venous valves at the thoracic inlet, pressure from the vena cava is not transmitted to the cerebral territory, thus maintaining cerebral perfusion during the phases of thoracic compression and thoracic decompression (33).

VENTRICULAR FIBRILLATION WAVE

As time passes in ventricular fibrillation, amplitude and frequency eventually decrease, ending in asystole. With CPR maneuvers and in relation to the generation of coronary flow, the opposite process occurs and the frequency and amplitude increase (48). Based on these characteristics, it is possible to predict the probability of terminating VF (ventricular fibrillation) and reestablishing cardiac activity with a shock.

POST-CARDIAC ARREST MANAGEMENT

Influences the final prognosis, due to the different post arrest management between hospitals there is great variability in prognosis. Resources needed for management include coronary catheterization, core body temperature management protocols, and expertise in neurologic prognostic assessment, in addition to the ability to manage a critically ill patient. When acute myocardial infarction is suspected, emergency coronary catheterization should be considered, especially when it is with ST-segment elevation and the patient should be taken to the catheterization room as soon as possible. According to experts, ventricular fibrillation can be considered an indicator of myocardial infarction and therefore coronary catheterization would be indicated. As for final management, patients need intensive therapy by trained personnel and should know all the problems that occur in the post-arrest as is the myocardial dysfunction that is usually transient, but can become severe, manage the cerebral ischemic injury and make the prognostic evolution with the ability to make decisions. Even with a prolonged period of neurological deficit, recovery may be complete. For this reason, an early prognosis should not be given and should wait for a period of at least 3 days once normal body temperature has been restored (33).

For CPR to be effective, it should be started early, and for this reason one of the most important fundamentals in its management is the time of initiation of CPR. The survival rate is a function of time, in Basic CPR should be applied within the first 4 minutes and advanced CPR within the first 8 minutes, reaching a survival rate of 43%; but if advanced CPR is delayed until 16 minutes and the survival rate is reduced to 10%. And there is a delay in basic CPR of > 4-5 min the probability of survival is improbable (30).

PRONOSTICO

Postanoxic encephalopathy occurs in 80% of patients who survive CRA who are unconscious during the first hour. Only approximately 20% of patients who suffer cardiac arrest manage to recover without sequelae, 50% after a year present moderate or severe cognitive deficits and 30% remain unconscious for a long time. The severity of the neurological symptoms after CPR will depend on the length of time that ischemia persists, the quality of CPR, the cardiac status before CPR and the hemodynamic situation after resuscitation. Recovery is also a function of depends on the time that patients are in coma, patients who are <12 hours in coma have a better recovery, while patients in coma > 1 week usually remain in a vegetative state due to laminar necrosis of the cortex where the function of the brain stem is preserved.

In the immediate clinical evaluation, patients with a good prognosis are those who take <25 min to recover spontaneous heartbeat, with an SBP (systolic blood pressure) > or = 90 mmHg and who are reactive or have spontaneous limb movements. However, studies have shown that it is impossible to predict who will develop irreversible neurological deficits during early assessment, as many patients often present with neurological deterioration in the first few minutes after spontaneous heartbeat recovery.

Advanced Life Support (ALS) Treatment Algorithm

Interventions that undoubtedly contribute to improved survival after cardiac arrest include rapid and effective bystander basic life support (BLS), high quality uninterrupted chest compressions and early defibrillation for VF/VST. The use of epinephrine has been shown to increase recovery of spontaneous circulation but not survival to discharge. Furthermore, there is a possibility that it may lead to worse long-term neurological survival. Also, evidence supporting advanced airway management during AVS remains limited (Soar et al. 2015) (30).

Soporte Vital Avanzado

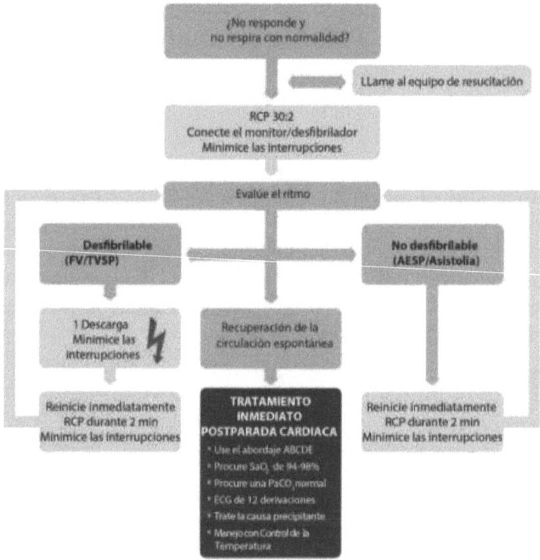

DURANTE RCP
- Asegure compresiones torácicas de alta calidad
- Minimice interrupciones de las compresiones
- Administre oxígeno
- Utilice capnografía con forma de onda
- Compresiones continuas cuando se haya asegurado la vía aérea
- Acceso vascular (intravenoso o intraóseo)
- Administre adrenalina cada 3-5 min
- Administre amiodarona después de 3 descargas

TRATAR LAS CAUSAS REVERSIBLES

Hipoxia	Trombosis – coronaria o pulmonar
Hipovolemia	Neumotórax a tensión
Hipo/hiperkalemia	Taponamiento cardíaco
Hipo/hipertermia	Tóxicos

Considerar
- Ecografía
- Compresiones torácicas mecánicas para facilitar traslado/tratamiento
- Coronariografía e intervención coronaria percutánea
- RCP extracorpórea

Ilustración 4. Algoritmo soporte vital avanzado tomado de: Guidelines for resuscitation 2015

Advanced life support algorithm taken from: Guidelines for resuscitation 2015

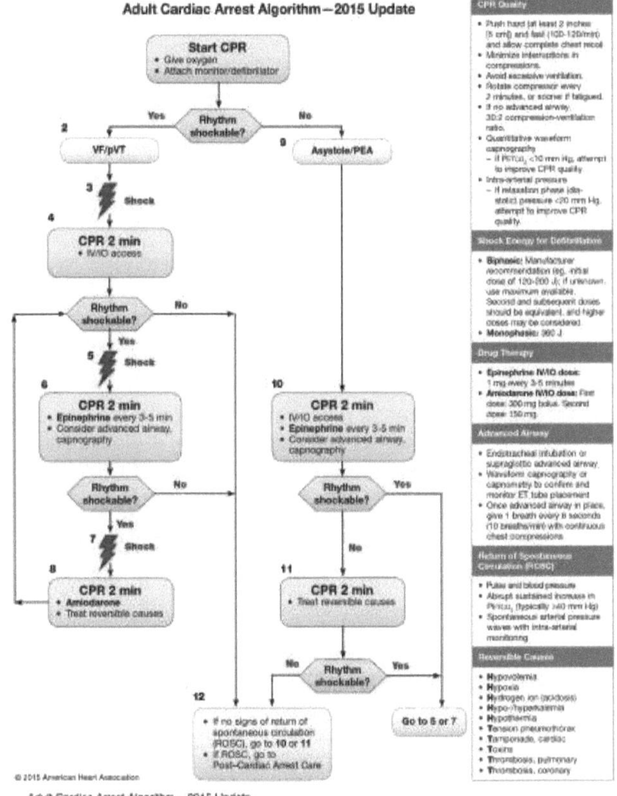

Ilustración 5 Algoritmo soporte vital avanzado, tomado de: AHA 2015

Advanced life support algorithm taken from: AHA 2015 (2015 American Heart Association Guidelines Update for Cardiopulmonary Resuscitation and Emergency Cardiovascular Care Circulation).

2.8. CARDIOPULMONARY RESUSCITATION IN THE GESTANTS

PHYSIOLOGICAL AND ANATOMICAL CHANGES DURING PREGNANCY

It is in the 20-32 OS (weeks of gestation) that gravida variations occur, which have repercussions on CPR manoeuvres (49).

Physiological modifications occur in the following systems:

- Respiratory
- Cardiovascular
- Hematology
- Gastrointestinal
- Renal (50)

At the cardiovascular system level there is an increase in CO (cardiac output) from 30-50% as a result of the increase in SV (systolic volume), and by the end of pregnancy this can reach up to 60%. (51) CPR manoeuvres should be performed while the caesarean section is being performed. There is an increase in maternal HR (heart rate) of 15-20 bpm, there is an increase in preload due to a 30-40% increase in plasma volume and a decrease in afterload due to an increase in progesterone or nitric oxide which are vasodilators and generate a decrease in peripheral vascular resistance. (52)

In relation to hematologic changes, there is an increase in plasma volume in the 30 OS, but these figures decrease until they normalize at the end of pregnancy, so there is usually dilution anemia, because there is a higher concentration of plasma volume and compared to the volume of red blood cells. (53) In addition, there is an elevation of fibrinogen levels, physiological leukocytosis and plateletopenia at the end of pregnancy (54). In the pregnant woman, when there are blood losses of >35%, signs of shock appear due to uteroplacental blood shunting. The main sign of hypotension is a drop in SBP (systolic blood pressure). (51)

At the gastrointestinal level, there is an increase in intragastric pressure and the function of the lower esophageal sphincter is altered according to data published in several articles related to physiological changes during pregnancy, there is an increase in intragastric pressure and incompetence of the lower esophageal sphincter and gastric emptying is slowed by the increase in uterine size and increased progesterone.(55) Intubation is necessary.

endotracheal in pregnant women because there is a risk of bronchial aspiration and regurgitation due to gastroesophageal reflux(56).

In the respiratory system, from 8 GS onwards, due to anatomical changes and hormonal effects, there are changes in lung capacities, volumes and ventilations. (53) According to the AHA (American Heart Association), during pregnancy the functional residual capacity decreases by 10-25%, because the uterus enlarges and the diaphragm rises. In the third trimester there is an increase in oxygen consumption of up to 20-33%. (52)

At the renal level, to regulate osmosis in the pregnant woman there is an increase in renal blood flow of 40% and an increase in the glomerular filtration rate, also this allows the elimination of fetal waste products. (54-66) According to the AHA this alteration of tubular function has a purpose and that is to avoid the loss of nutrients necessary for the fetus such as amino acids and glucose. (52)

MAIN CAUSES OF PCR IN PREGNANT WOMEN

The pregnant woman can suffer from the causes of a non-pregnant woman and add causes of CRP, that is why it is determined that the etiology in pregnant women is multicausal: (57)

Obstetric causes:	Non-obstetric causes
✓ Bleeding ✓ Preeclampsia ✓ HELLP Syndrome ✓ Amniotic fluid embolism ✓ Peripartum cardiomyopathy ✓ Anesthetic complications	✓ Pulmonary thromboembolism ✓ Septic shock ✓ Cardiovascular disease ✓ Endocrine disorders ✓ Collagen diseases ✓ Trauma

TABLE. Causes of CRP in pregnant women

"According to an article published by the Cuban Journal of Obstetrics and Gynecology on the impact of obstetric hemorrhage on maternal morbidity, it has been shown that hemorrhage is the most significant complication of pregnancy, while the Catalan Society of Anesthesiology and Resuscitation warns that hemorrhage constitutes 25% of cases of maternal death in developed countries" (55),

PECULIARITIES OF RESUSCITATION MANEUVERS IN THE SEQUENCE OF BASIC AND ADVANCED CPR IN PREGNANT WOMEN

According to the AHA, resuscitation in pregnant women is the same as CPR in adults, with some peculiarities in the particular maneuvers:

BASIC LIFE SUPPORT IN PREGNANT WOMEN

Cardiac massage technique in pregnant women:

When the victim is a pregnant woman, it is a priority to perform high-quality CPR and remove aortocaval pressure. If the fundus is found at or above the umbilicus, the uterus should be shifted to the left to remove the aortocaval compression that occurs during chest compressions. When there is maternal trauma, with the mother's pulse absent for a long time or with non-viable survival and no response to resuscitation, delivery should not be delayed by perimortem caesarean section, 4 minutes after CPR and without success to resuscitation efforts. (35)

According to AHA recommendations, chest compressions in gestation are performed on a firm surface area, at a rate of 100 to 120 bpm and at a depth of 5 cm (2 inches); allowing complete re-expansion of the chest before each compression; the compression/ventilation ratio is 30:2; it is important to limit interruptions to no more than 10 seconds. (52)

Aortocaval compression syndrome occurs when performing chest compressions. When the pregnant woman is placed in the supine decubitus position, the aorta artery and inferior vena cava are compressed, which causes a decrease in venous return and CO, manifesting itself in the clinic as hypotension, syncope in the supine decubitus position and bradycardia; to avoid this situation, the pregnant woman should be placed in left lateral decubitus with a 30° angle of inclination and in this way aortocaval compression is reduced. (58)

The AHA recommends left lateral hand displacement of the uterus during resuscitation to decrease aortocaval compression, taking into account that the uterus should be palpable above the uterus or at the level of the umbilicus. (52)

As for the airway, the basic life support algorithm of the AHA is used as a reference, which consists of opening the airway by means of the forehead-chin maneuver if there is no cervical injury, since in this case mandibular traction is performed; 100% oxygen is administered at a flow rate greater than or equal to 15 L/min and the compression/ventilation ratio 30:2 with bag-mask. (49)

If rhythm alterations such as VF (ventricular fibrillation) and PSVT (pulseless ventricular tachycardia) are present, which are the defibrillable rhythms, the shock should be performed. (4-8-9) According to the AHA, for defibrillation, the energy required for CRP in pregnant women is the same as that of a non-pregnant adult, 300 Joules in a monophasic rhythm and 200 Joules in a biphasic rhythm, since there are no modifications that intervene in the flow of the transmyocardial energy current. (51)

ADVANCED LIFE SUPPORT IN PREGNANT WOMEN

According to official guidelines the resuscitation team should follow the maternal CPR algorithm. (52)

<table>
<tr><td>Advanced Life Support (ALS) Algorithm</td></tr>
<tr><td>

1. Evaluate rhythm: monitoring.
2. Defibrillation: if Ventricular Fibrillation (VF) or Pulseless Ventricular Tachycardia (PVT).
3. Orotracheal intubation: if not possible, use alternative supra glottic VA devices.
4. CPR technique: quality chest compressions at a rate of 100-120/min. Minimize interruptions. 8-10 ventilations/min once VA is isolated.
5. Intravenous line: cannulate peripheral venous line (PVL) first. If this is not possible, cannulate intraosseous route.
6. Drugs:
√ Adrenaline 1 milligram (mg) intravenous (IV) every 3-5 minutes.
√ Amiodarone 300mg IV bolus after 3rd shock in defibrillable rhythms.
7. Correct reversible causes

</td></tr>
</table>

TABLE. Algorithm of Advanced Life Support (ALS) (2019) obtained from: *"Manual Therapeutic" Ediciones Universidad de Salamanca. (23)*

It is necessary to activate and notify not only the maternal CPR team but also the neonatal CPR team, and to have the Caesarean section team ready in case of emergency. The ALS team will be in charge of airway management until endotracheal intubation to avoid serious complications; a 6-7 mm diameter tube is recommended; if intubation fails twice, a supra glottic device should be placed; and if ventilation with a mask is not effective, cricothyrotomy should be performed (52).

An intravenous access must be placed above the diaphragm for drug administration. Drug treatment of CRA in pregnant women is the same as in adults. In pregnant women with tachycardia and refractory ventricular fibrillation who do not respond to defibrillation, the drug of choice is amiodarone and as a second option epinephrine (1 mg IV or intraosseous every 5 min). (59)

According to the AHA, when there is a response after 4 minutes of CPR, the team should prepare for emergency caesarean section (in pregnant women with > 20 OS), it is important to keep the uterus lateralized to the left until the fetus is born. When uterine evacuation occurs, venous return increases, aortocaval compression decreases and CPR is effective. (60)

2.9. LEGAL FRAMEWORK

It is of great interest to note that in order for a physician to join the Ministry of Public Health, he or she has a series of responsibilities that must be fulfilled and that are expressed in his or her contract, but it is equally important to be aware that all public servants have the right to be trained by their employer. In this case, the Ministry of Public Health must schedule and carry out all the courses that are requested so that the servant is up-to-date, and if it does not have personnel who can carry out the training, they can look for an entity outside the public network to do so.

Art. 195.- On education and training.

- The subsystem of training and education for the public sector constitutes the set of policies and procedures established to regulate public service career studies in order to achieve the training, competencies and skills, which in some way may be performed by public servants in accordance with the occupational profiles and requirements established in the positions of an organization, and thus may affirm the achievement of the portfolio of institutional products and services, its planning and the objectives established in the National Development Plan. (61)

Art. 196.- The formative and educational objectives.

-    The objectives of the training and education will be as follows:

•   To count with servers and servants with technical, professional training and education or with fourth level specializations related to institutional and national needs and objectives;
•   Promote the generation of scientific knowledge through applied research in fields of national interest; and,
•   Generate the development of capacities, abilities and skills in public servants.

Art. 197.- Those responsible for training and professional training.

- Training and education will be the responsibility of an inter-institutional committee composed of the following institutions: National Secretariat for Planning and Development, Ministry of Labour Relations and Institute of Higher National Studies, who will establish the national policy for public sector training and education.

Technical standards shall be issued through the Ministry of Labour Relations for the application of its provisions, without prejudice to others that may be issued for this purpose. (61)

Article 204 - Ecuadorian Professional Training Service.

-    The Ecuadorian Vocational Training Service will form a fundamental part of the Training Networks and will be the body in charge of the technical institutions, operationalization of the capacity of non-professionals, companies, entities and organizations established within the scope of the LOSEP, in the areas of its competence. (61)

Article 205 - Specialized training services.

-    The UATH, in accordance with the policies, rules and instruments established by the Ministry of Labour Relations, shall be empowered to contract specialized training services with legal or natural persons from both the private and public sectors that are qualified by the Ministry of Labour Relations. (61)

Article 208.- Training and updating of knowledge of public servants for the performance of institutional services.

-      When a public servant who has obtained a free appointment or has been removed from office travels to carry out official training tasks and, above all, to update his or her knowledge at conferences, visits, meetings, observation within or outside the country, he or she shall be granted secondment with remuneration, receiving per diem, subsistence, travel and transportation expenses for the duration of the secondment from the date of departure to the date of his or her return. (51)

2.10.   Research variable DEPENDENTS

- PCR Identification
- Chest compression
- CPR Pregnant women
- Airway Management
- ventilation
- Early defibrillation
- Drugs used in CPR
- Pediatric CPR

Knowledge of emergency health personnel about cardiopulmonary resuscitation.

INDEPENDENT

Characterization of variables: age, sex, length of work experience, profession, participation in CPR training and participation in CPR maneuvers in real situations.

3. METHODOLOGICAL FRAMEWORK

3.6. CHARACTERIZATION OF THE WORK AREA

The present study was carried out in Ecuador, in the Province of Los Ríos, Cantón Quevedo, Zonal 5, at the Hospital Sagrado Corazón de Jesús in the city of Quevedo, located at Avenida Guayacanes 400 and AV. Walter Andrade. It is a basic hospital that corresponds to the second level of health care belonging to the health district 12D03 Mocache-Quevedo.

3.7. UNIVERSE AND SAMPLE UNIVERSE

Taking data of human resources of the health personnel of the emergency area of Sacred Heart of Jesus Hospital, which are included in this study are:

- General Emergency Resident Physicians: 25
- General Emergency Nursing Graduates: 5
- Resident physicians of the gynecological-obstetric emergency area: 5
- Emergency Obstetrics/Gynecology/Gynecology and Obstetrics Emergency Nurses: 5

SAMPLE

The population described above of the health professionals of the Sacred Heart of Jesus Hospital in the emergency area is 40 people, of which we were able to evaluate the 40 people who were available and willing to take the surveys for the research.

3.8. ELIGIBILITY REQUIREMENTS

Inclusion Criteria	Exclusion Criteria
- members of the general emergency and gynecology-obstetrics area team - resident doctors and nursing graduates. - Who voluntarily agree to participate in the study.	- Staff who do not wish to participate in the study - personnel who are not part of the emergency area.

3.9. FEASIBILITY

The research work carried out was viable in the first place because of the approval previously granted by the authorities of the University of Guayaquil, and the directors of the Hospital Sagrado Corazón de Jesús who authorized the realization of the research. We would also like to thank the health personnel of the emergency area who collaborated with their participation in carrying out the surveys.

3.10.   RESEARCH DESIGN

The research work is of quantitative approach, non-experimental design, cross-sectional and the method is observational.

3.11.   HUMAN AND PHYSICAL RESOURCES Human Resources

- Researchers
- Thesis tutor
- Thesis reviewer
- Hospital Director
- Emergency Physicians and Emergency Department Graduates

Physical Resources

- Computer
- Printer
- Sheets
- Cellular
- Notebooks
- Medical Journals
- Internet access
- Medical publishers

3.12. EVALUATION OR DATA COLLECTION INSTRUMENTS.

DATA

For the data collection of the present investigation, the survey technique was used and the instrument was a questionnaire, which contains statements that are referred to a series of activities that have been selected in response to the indicators, in which the health professional of the emergency area of the Sacred Heart of Jesus Hospital must respond.

This instrument was subjected to the reliability test, because it was created exclusively for the research.

3.13. METHODOLOGY FOR THE ANALYSIS OF RESULTS

Once the data were obtained, they were processed by means of statistical packages after the elaboration of the code table, thus assigning the corresponding value of 1 (correct question) and 0 (incorrect question) to the answer.

All this in order to then be presented in graphs or statistical tables for analysis and interpretation considering the background and the theoretical framework, which help us with the explanation of the results and conclusions.

3.14. BIOETHICAL CONSIDERATIONS

The information obtained for this study was provided by conducting a survey of resident physicians and nursing graduates in the emergency area of the Sacred Heart of Jesus Hospital, after the request was approved by Dr. Cando Palma Alex Orlando, head of the emergency area.

For the execution of the questionnaire, informed consent was requested in writing from the resident physicians and nursing graduates in the emergency area. Likewise, privacy will be respected at all times through the anonymity of the research subjects.

Description and operationalization of the variables

variable	conceptual definition	operational definition	dimensions		measurement scale n
Knowledge of basic and advanced cardiopulmonary resuscitation and advanced	Collected information on basic and advanced cardiopulmonary resuscitation to restore vital functions in the event of cardiopulmonary arrest. cardiorespiratory arrest	Information available to health personnel in the emergency health workers have about cardiopulmonary resuscitation onary cardiopulmonary resuscitation (CPR), lo that will allow them to be applied during care of the patient presenting cardiopulmonary arrest.	General	Definition of Cardiac Arrest * Types of cardiorespiratory arrest Signs and Symptoms of Cardiac Arrest Definition of resuscitation Chain of Survival CPR Sequence * High quality CPR CPR in	Ordinal scale *High *Medium *Low
			Management of chest compressions	Depth Time Frequency location Compression of compression	Ordinal scale *High *Medium *Low
			Airway Management	Cause of Airway Obstruction Method to clear the airway with cervical problem Method of clearing airway without cervical problem	Ordinal scale *High *Medium *Low

			Ventilation	Compression/ventilation ratio Time Technique	Ordinal scale *High *Medium *Low
			Automated External Defibrillation	Technique *Application	Ordinal scale *High *Medium *Low
			Drugs used in Basic Life Support	Dose frequency Route of administration	Ordinal scale *High *Medium *Low

Variable	Definition	Type of variable	Scale	Indicator
Sex	Male organic condition or female	qualitative	Male Female	Percentage
Age	Time the person has lived in completed years, up to the time of the survey. data	quantitative	Years completed	average
Length of work experience	Time practicing the profession until the date of collection of data	Quantitative	Years of work experience	average
Participating in CPR maneuvers in real life situations	Witnessing and assisting a cardiac arrest	quantitative	Number of events	average

Participation in CPR trainings	Attended CPR training or courses in the last 3 years	quantitative	• Basic CPR • Advanced CPR • None	percentage
Professional is health	Usual activity of a person for which he/she has prepared himself/herself	qualitative	List of health professionals	percentage

4. RESULTS AND DISCUSSION

At the end of the data collection through the questionnaire, the data were processed and represented in graphs and statistical tables, in order to achieve a better analysis and understanding.

4.6. Results

At the conclusion of the research work on basic and advanced cardiopulmonary resuscitation in the emergency area of the Sacred Heart of Jesus Hospital in the city of Quevedo, with a sample of 40 people of whom 30 are medical residents and 10 are nursing graduates, surveys containing 20 questions were conducted.

The Gaussian bell was used to classify the CPR knowledge of the health care personnel in the emergency area (resident physicians and nursing graduates) and it was divided into 3 categories:
HIGH, MEDIUM AND LOW.

Number of questions: 20

Arithmetic average: 10
Standard deviation: 6

We set the values for a and b a = 10 - (6 x 0.75) = 5.4 ≈ 5

b = 10 + (6 x 0.75) = 14.54 ≈ 15

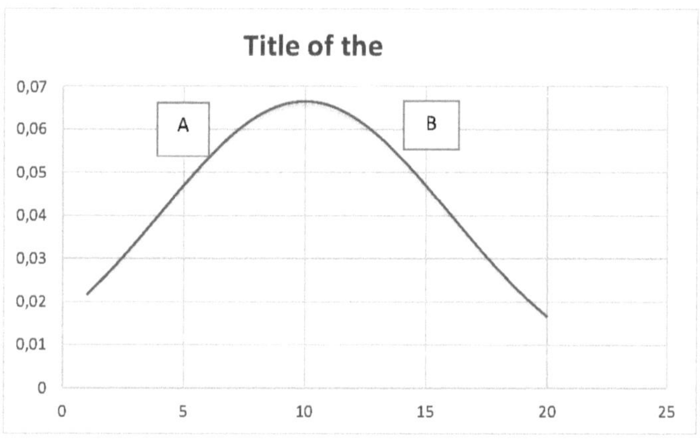

DEMOGRAPHIC VARIABLES:

Table 1 Sex and age of health personnel at Sacred Heart of Jesus Hospital.

SEX	FEMALE		MALE		TOTAL	
AGE	N°	%	N°	%	N°	%
27-37 years old	22	55	7	17,5	29	72,5
38-48 years old	5	12,5	1	2,5	6	15
49-59 years old	2	5	1	2,5	3	7,5
60 years and older	2	5	0	0	2	5
TOTAL	31	77,5	9	22,5	40	100

SOURCE: DATABASE ELABORATED BY: AUTHORS

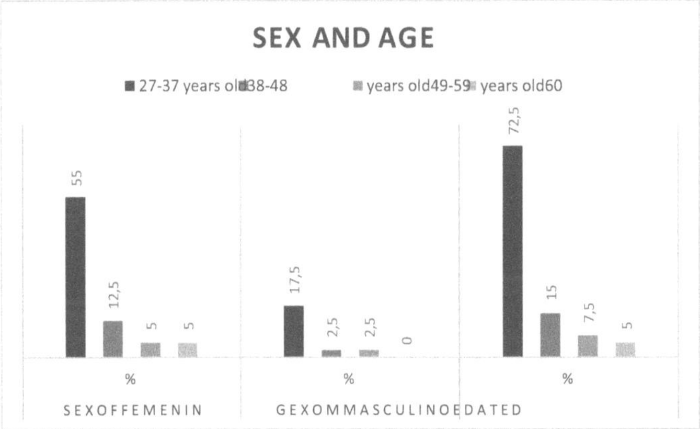

Graph 1 Sex and age of health personnel at Sacred Heart of Jesus Hospital.

- **Interpretation:** Sex: Analyzing the data obtained with the sex variable we find that 22.5% represent the male sex and 77.5% represent the female sex, **the participants have a ratio of 3.4:1 with the female sex being greater**. This leads us to think that in recent years the number of female professionals has increased.
- **Interpretation**: Age: Participants ranged in age from.
27 to 62 years of age, **we observe that the majority of the personnel represented with 72.5% are between the ages of 27-37 years**, followed by

15% between 38-48 years, 7.5% between 49-59 years and 5% with 60 years or more.

Table 2 Distribution by training in cardiopulmonary resuscitation received in the last 3 years by health personnel in the emergency area of the hospital sagrado corazón de Jesús.

TRAINING ABOUT CPR	NUMBER OF PROFESSIONALS	%
I RECEIVE	30	75%
NO RECEIPT	10	25%
TOTAL	40	100%

SOURCE: DATABASE ELABORATED BY: AUTHORS

CHART No.

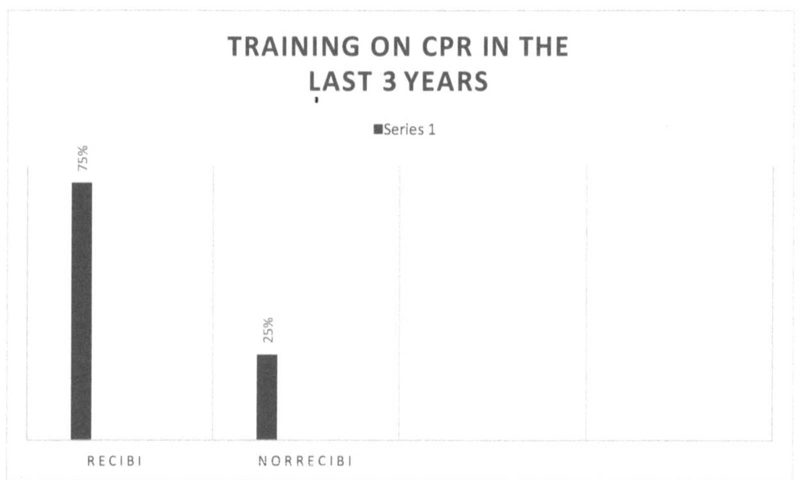

Graph 2 Distribution by training in cardiopulmonary resuscitation received in the last 3 years by health personnel in the emergency area of the hospital sagrado corazón de Jesús.

- **Interpretation:** Completion of CPR course is very important for all health personnel as they should be ready to provide support if required. Analyzing the data obtained with the variable CPR training **in the last 3 years, we found that 75% had received training** and 25% had not.

Table 3 Distribution by type of training (basic/advanced CPR) received by health personnel in the emergency area of the hospital sagrado corazón de Jesús.

TYPE OF TRAINING	N°	%
BASIC	9	22%
BASIC AND ADVANCED	21	53%
NONE	10	25%
TOTAL	40	100%

SOURCE: DATABASE ELABORATED BY: AUTHORS

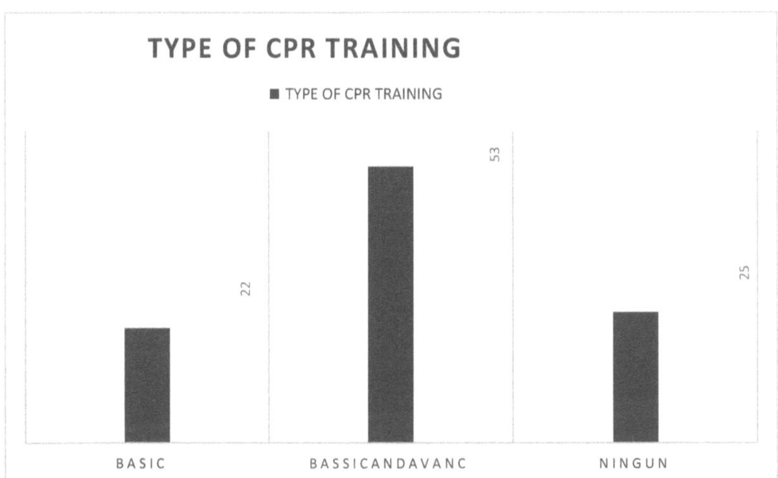

Graph 3 Distribution by type of training (basic/advanced CPR) received by health personnel in the emergency area of the hospital sagrado corazón de Jesús.

Interpretation: If we analyze the percentage that received training in the last 3 years (30), we observe that 22% received training in Basic CPR, **53% received training in Basic/Advanced CPR** and **25% did not receive training in Basic or Advanced CPR.**

Table 4 Distribution by time of work experience of health personnel in the emergency area of the Sacred Heart of Jesus Hospital.

TIME OF EXPERIENCE LABOR	N°	%
1-5 years	22	55
6-10 years	7	17,5
11-15 years old	6	15
16-20 years old	3	7,5
More than 20 years	2	5
TOTAL	40	100

SOURCE: DATABASE ELABORATED BY: AUTHORS

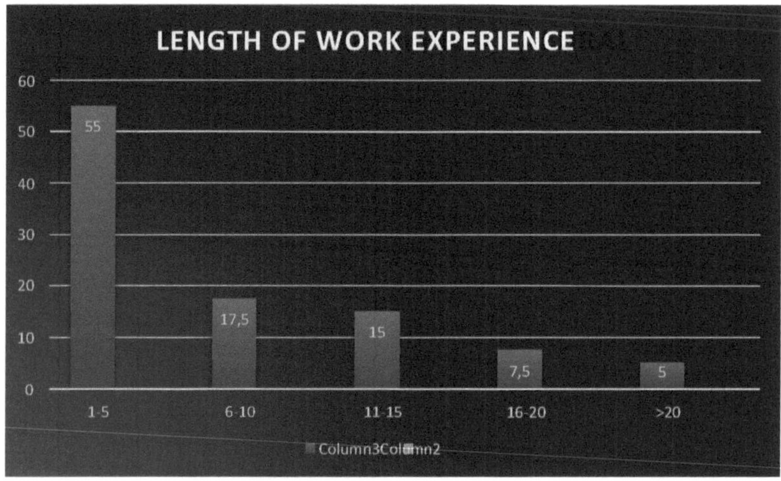

Graph 4 Distribution by time of work experience of health personnel in the emergency area of the Sacred Heart of Jesus Hospital.

Interpretation: Analyzing the variable in terms of time of work experience, we observe that **the majority of health personnel have between 1-5 years of work experience, represented by 55%,** followed by 17.5% between 6-10 years, 15% between 11-15 years, 7.5% between 16-20 years, and 5% of personnel with 20 years or more.

Table 5 Distribution by profession of health personnel in the emergency area of the Sacred Heart of Jesus Hospital.

PROFESSION	N°	%
General Emergency Resident Physician	25	62,5
Gynecological Emergency Resident Physician obstetric	5	12,5
General Emergency Nurse Practitioner	5	12,5
Licensed emergency gynecological nurse. obstetric	5	12,5
TOTAL	40	100

SOURCE: DATABASE ELABORATED BY: AUTHORS

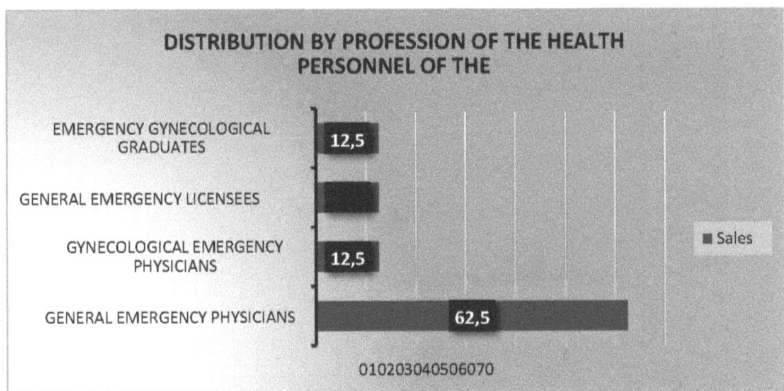

Graph 5 Distribution by profession of health personnel in the emergency area of the Sacred Heart of Jesus Hospital.

Interpretation: The inclusion criteria for our study included all health personnel in the emergency area, **62.5% of whom were general emergency physicians, which is the majority of the staff**; 12.5% were emergency obstetrics and gynecology physicians; 12.5% were general emergency physicians; 12.5% were emergency obstetrics and gynecology graduates; and 12.5% were emergency obstetrics and gynecology graduates.

Correct	N°	%
11	1	
12	1	2,5
13	6	15
14	6	15
15	6	15
16	8	20
17	9	22,5
18	1	2,5
19	2	5
TOTAL	40	100

RANGE	N°	%	LEVEL
0 a 4	0	0	BAJO
5 a 14	14	35	MEDIO
15 a 20	26	65	ALTO
TOTAL	40	100	

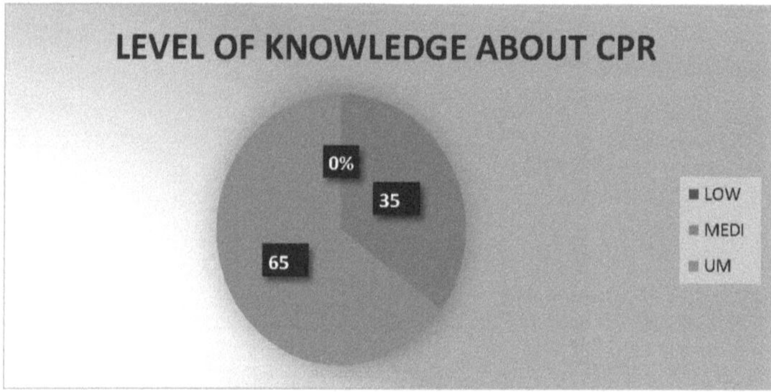

Graph 6 Level of knowledge of basic and advanced cardiopulmonary resuscitation among health personnel in the emergency area of the Hospital Sagrado Corazón de Jesús.

Interpretation: In graph x on the level of knowledge of the health professional on basic and advanced cardiopulmonary resuscitation, it can be seen that the health personnel in the emergency area surveyed (40) in 100%, we observe that **65% (26 professionals) have high knowledge, emphasizing that it is the highest average**. Thirty-five percent (14 professionals) have a medium level of knowledge and 0% have a low level of knowledge.

Table 7 Level of knowledge of the variable CPR identification and conditions for CPR among health personnel in the emergency area of the Hospital Sagrado Corazón de Jesús.

Number of correct questions	N°	%
1	0	0
2	2	5
3	4	10
4	16	40
5	18	45
total, participants	40	100

RANGE	N°	%	LEVEL
0 a 1	0	0	BAJO
2 a 3	6	15	MEDIO
4 a 5	34	85	ALTO
total	40	100	

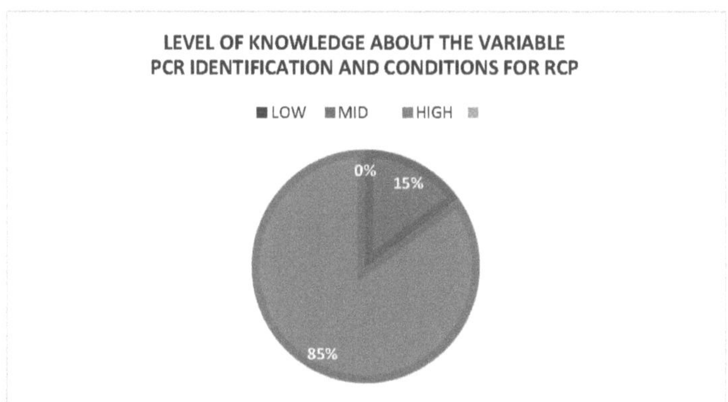

Graph 7 Level of knowledge of the variable CPR identification and conditions for CPR among health personnel in the emergency area of the Hospital Sagrado Corazón de Jesús.

Interpretation: In graph 7 regarding the level of knowledge of the health professional on identification of CRA and conditions for CPR, we observe that **85% (34 professionals) present a high level of knowledge**, being the highest; and 15% present a medium level of knowledge and 0% present a low knowledge.

Table 8 Level of knowledge of the variable chest compressions among health personnel in the emergency area of the Hospital Sagrado Corazón de Jesús.

Correct questions	N°	%
1	0	0
2	9	22,5
3	18	45
4	13	32,5
total	40	100

RANGE	N°	%	LEVEL
0 a 1	0	0	BAJO
2 a 3	27	67	MEDIO
4.	13	33	ALTO
TOTAL	40	100	

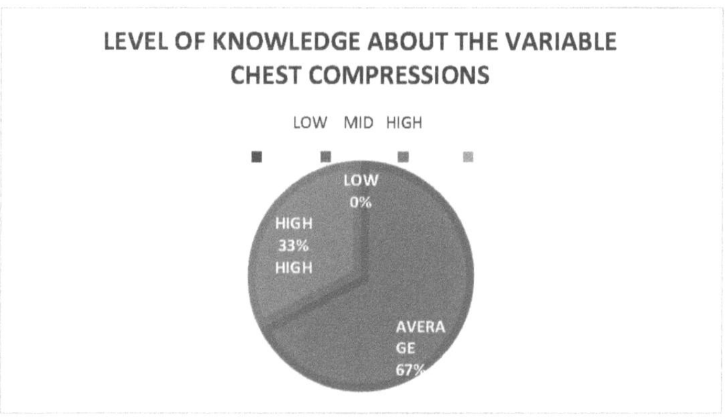

Graph 8 Level of knowledge of the variable chest compressions among health personnel in the emergency area of the Hospital Sagrado Corazón de Jesús.

Interpretation: In graph 8 regarding the level of knowledge of the health professional on application of chest compressions, we observe that **67% (27 professionals) present a medium level of knowledge, being the highest percentage.** Thirty-three percent have a high level of knowledge and 0% have a low level of knowledge.

Table 9 Level of knowledge of the variable airway management among health personnel in the emergency area of the Hospital Sagrado Corazón de Jesús.

questions correct	N°	%
0	1	2,5
1	8	20
2	22	55
3	9	22,5
total	40	100

RANGE	N°	%	LEVEL
0 a 1	9	22	BAJO
2.	22	56	MEDIO
3.	9	22	ALTO
TOTAL	40	100	

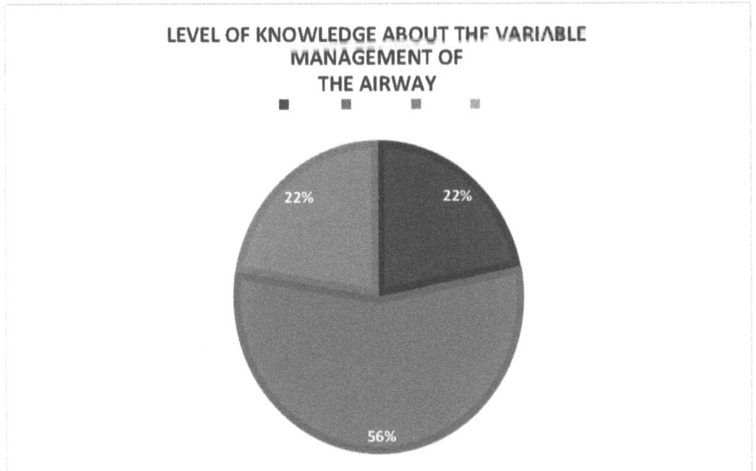

Graph 9 Level of knowledge of the variable airway management among health personnel in the emergency area of the Hospital Sagrado Corazón de Jesús.

Interpretation: In graph 9 on health professional's level of knowledge on airway management, it can be seen that **56% (22 professionals) have medium level of knowledge, being the highest percentage**. Twenty-two percent (22%) have a high level of knowledge and 22% have a low level of knowledge.

Table 10 Level of knowledge of the variable ventilation among health personnel in the emergency area of the Hospital Sagrado Corazón de Jesús.

Questions correct	N°	%
1	4	10
2	14	35
3	22	55
total	40	100

RANGE	N°	%	LEVEL
0 a 1	4	10	BAJO
2.	14	35	MEDIO
3.	22	55	ALTO
TOTAL	40	100	

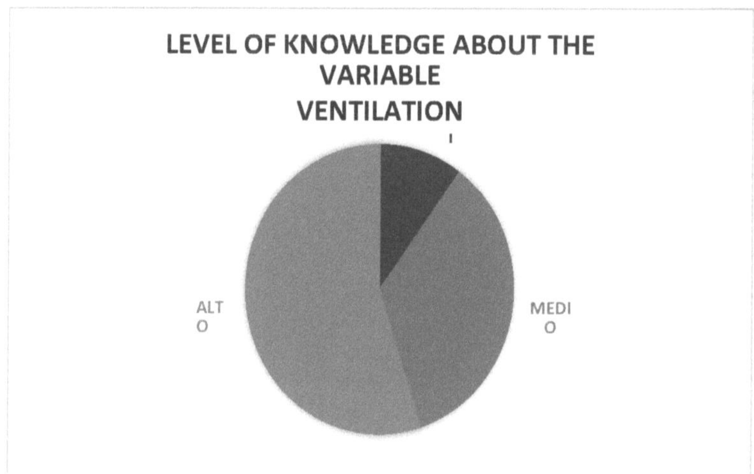

Graph 10 Level of knowledge of the variable ventilation among health personnel in the emergency area of the Hospital Sagrado Corazón de Jesús.

Interpretation: In graph 10 on level of knowledge of the health professional about ventilation, it can be observed that **55% (22 professionals) present a high level of knowledge,** emphasizing that it is the highest percentage. Thirty-five percent have a medium level of knowledge and 10% have a low level of knowledge.

Table 11 Level of knowledge of the variable early defibrillation among health personnel in the emergency area of the Hospital Sagrado Corazón de Jesús.

Number of correct questions	N°	%
1	14	35
2	26	65
total	40	100

RANGE	N°	%	LEVEL
0.	0	0	BAJO
1.	14	35	MEDIO
2.	26	65	ALTO
TOTAL	40	100	

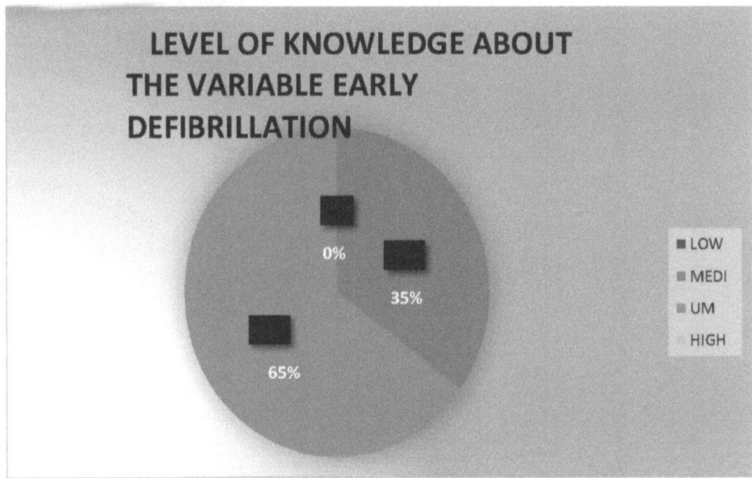

Graph 11 Level of knowledge of the variable early defibrillation among health personnel in the emergency area of the Hospital Sagrado Corazón de Jesús.

Interpretation: In graph 11 on level of knowledge of health professional on early defibrillation, it is observed that **65% (26 professionals) present a high level of knowledge, being the highest**. Thirty-five percent (35%) have a medium level of knowledge and 0% have a low level of knowledge.

Table 12 Level of knowledge of the variable drug administration among health personnel in the emergency area of the Sacred Heart of Jesus Hospital.

N° right questions	N°	%
0	2	5
1	8	20
2	23	57,5
3	7	17,5
Total	40	100

RANGE	N°	%	LEVEL
0-1	10	25	BAJO
2.	23	57,5	MEDIO
3.	7	17,5	ALTO
TOTAL	40	100	

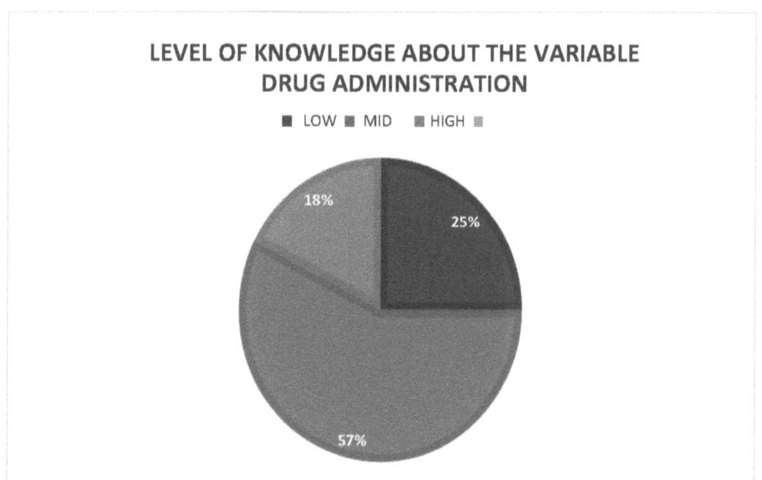

Graph 12 Level of knowledge of the variable drug administration among health personnel in the emergency area of the Sacred Heart of Jesus Hospital.

Interpretation: In graph 12 on level of knowledge of health professional on drug administration, it is observed that **57% (23 professionals) present a medium level of knowledge, being the highest**. Twenty-five percent have a low level of knowledge and 18% have a high level of knowledge.

Table 13 Level of knowledge of basic and advanced CPR according to years of work experience from 1 to 5 years among health personnel in the emergency area of the hospital sagrado corazón de Jesús.

Years of experience	NO	%
FROM 1 TO 5 YEARS	16	73
	6	27
TOTAL	22	100

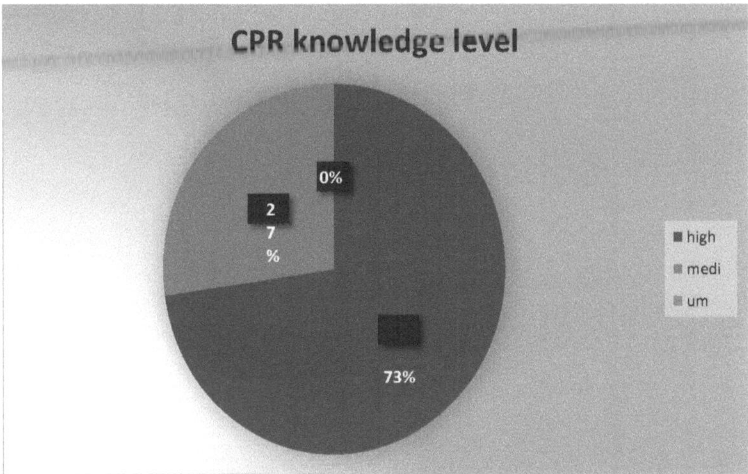

Graph 13 Level of knowledge of basic and advanced CPR according to years of work experience of more than 20 years among health personnel in the emergency area of the hospital sagrado corazón de Jesús.

Interpretation: In relation to the knowledge of basic and advanced cardiopulmonary resuscitation of the staff in relation to their years of experience from **1 to 5 years (22 professionals), it is found that 73% (16 professionals) have high knowledge**, and 27% (6 professionals) have medium knowledge.

Table 14 Level of knowledge of basic and advanced CPR according to years of work experience from 6 to 10 years among health personnel in the emergency area of the hospital sagrado corazón de Jesús.

	NO	%
FROM 6 TO 10 YEARS OLD	3	43
	4	57
TOTAL	7	100

CPR knowledge level

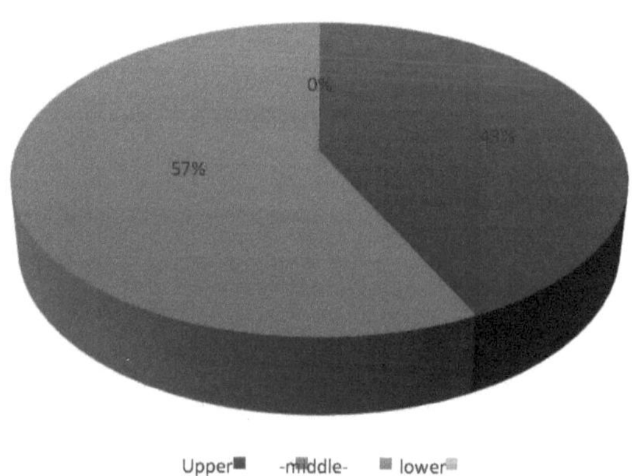

Graph 14 Level of knowledge of basic and advanced CPR according to years of work experience from 6 to 10 years among health personnel in the emergency area of the hospital sagrado corazón de Jesús.

Interpretation: In relation to the knowledge of basic CPR of the staff in relation to their years of experience **from 6 to 10 years (7 professionals), it is found that 57% (4 professionals) have medium knowledge,** and 43% (3 professionals) have high knowledge.

Table 15 Level of knowledge of basic and advanced CPR according to years of work experience from 11 to 15 years among health personnel in the emergency area of the hospital sagrado corazón de Jesús.

	N0	%
FROM 11 TO 15	4	67
YEARS OLD	2	33
TOTAL	6	100

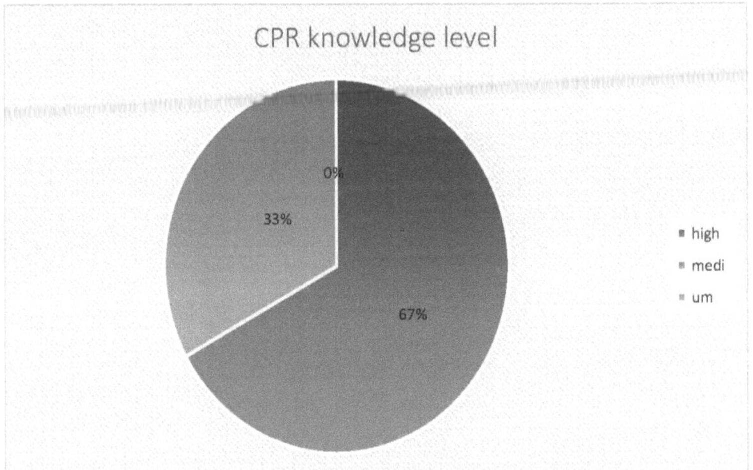

Graph 15 Level of knowledge of basic and advanced CPR according to years of work experience from 11 to 15 years among health personnel in the emergency area of the hospital sagrado corazón de Jesús.

Interpretation: In relation to the knowledge of basic and advanced cardiopulmonary resuscitation of health personnel in relation to their years of experience from **11 to 15 years (6 professionals), it is found that 67% (4 professionals) have high knowledge**, and 33% (2 professionals) have medium knowledge.

Table 16 Level of knowledge of basic and advanced CPR according to years of work experience from 16 to 20 years among health personnel in the emergency area of the hospital sagrado corazón de Jesús.

	NO	%
FROM 16 TO 20	2	67
YEARS OLD	1	33
TOTAL	3	100

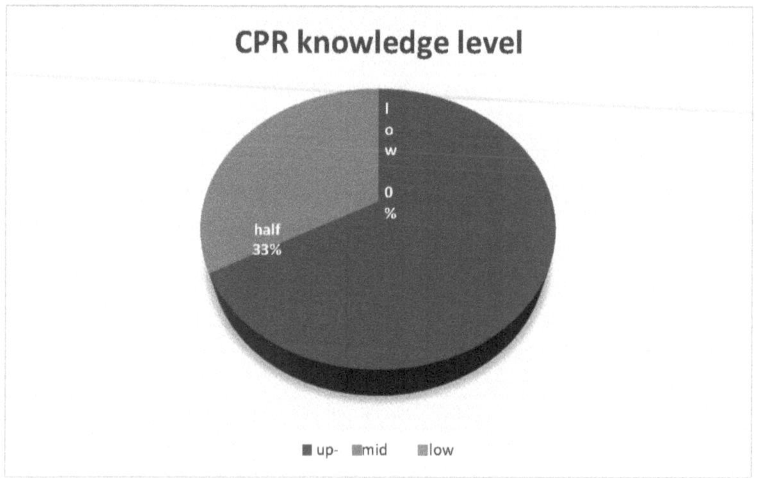

Graph 16 Level of knowledge of basic and advanced CPR according to years of work experience from 16 to 20 years of age among health personnel in the emergency area of the hospital sagrado corazón de Jesús.

Interpretation: In relation to the knowledge of basic and advanced cardiopulmonary resuscitation of the staff in relation to their years of experience from **16 to 20 years (3 professionals), it is found that 67% (2 professionals) have high knowledge**, and 33% (1 professionals) have medium knowledge.

Table 17 Level of knowledge of basic and advanced CPR according to years of work experience of more than 20 years among health personnel in the emergency area of the hospital sagrado corazón de Jesús.

	NO	%
OVER 20 YEARS OF EXPERIENCE	1	50
	1	50
TOTAL	2	100

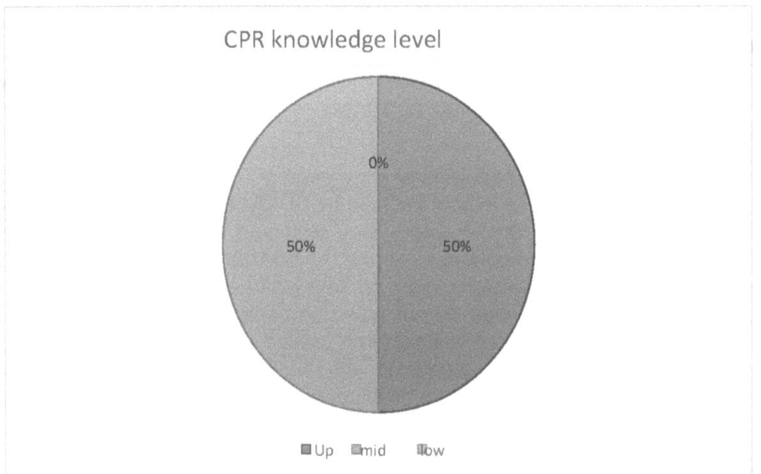

Graph 17 Level of knowledge of basic and advanced CPR according to years of work experience of more than 20 years among health personnel in the emergency area of the hospital sagrado corazón de Jesús.

Interpretation: In relation to the knowledge of basic and advanced cardiopulmonary resuscitation of health personnel in relation to their years of experience of **more than 20 years (2 professionals), it is found that 50% (1 professional) have high knowledge, and 50% (1 professional) have medium knowledge.**

4.7. DISCUSSION

It is essential in hospitals that all health professionals have adequate and updated knowledge about basic and advanced cardiopulmonary resuscitation, especially in the most critical areas. Emphasizing that the emergency team are the first to attend to victims of cardiac arrest obtaining interesting results. For this reason the AHA has developed protocols, which are updated every 5 years to provide timely care. It is essential that health care personnel be trained in CPR. Resident physicians must have the knowledge and skills to apply CPR techniques, since they are part of the chain of survival. We agree with the Accreditation Council for Medical Education in the United States which has established that CPR knowledge and skills are very necessary and indispensable for health personnel who graduate from their profession (16), something that does not occur in Ecuador, and this is what led us to evaluate the level of knowledge of health personnel in a critical area such as the emergency area.

In our study we obtained a high level of knowledge of CPR represented by 65%. We agree with the study carried out in Quito by Dr. Cynthia Cabrera Jurado and Dr. Christopher Cedillo Carrión, where they observed that 79% of physicians and nurses know the importance of the immediate and timely response protocol. (51) In CPR, all actions must be timely and effective; personnel with an average level of knowledge do not have the capacity to reverse CPR and can make many errors that can limit recovery, cause sequelae and even lead to death. However, there are discrepancies with studies carried out in Peru, such as the study by Reyes, where it was concluded that the health personnel in the Emergency Department have an average level of knowledge of CPR (14). In another study by Carmen Escriba Mendoza and Wilberth Sulca Barrón, the highest percentage of health professionals (61.1%) had average knowledge of basic CPR and only 38.9% performed CPR correctly (77). (77) In the study carried out by German Aranzábal-Alegría, Araseli Verastegui-Día, it was concluded that the level of knowledge was low; this should be considered in order to generate policies for updating and continuous education, so that health personnel are prepared in theory and practice, thus avoiding complications and deaths. (75) In the study carried out in Paraguay by Aldo López-González, Walter Delgado, 83.7% presented an unsatisfactory level, not answering correctly at least 17 questions of the questionnaire. (76)

Regarding the level of knowledge about the variable identification of cardiac arrest, it was found that the majority of health personnel 85% have a high level of knowledge. In agreement with the study done in Quito by Dr. Cynthia Cabrera Jurado, Dr. Christopher Cedillo Carrión, 88.9% have a satisfactory level of knowledge in the question that assessed the identification of CRA "if the professional can identify an arrest in time, he/she can start the resuscitation with less time delay which gives a good prognosis for the patient". (51) There is a discrepancy in the study conducted by Dr. Indira Gisella Reyes Moran since the majority of health personnel present a medium level with 52.3% and a relevant minority 30.2% a low level. (14) It is essential to recognize CPR since it is the key to initiate CPR. Personnel should know the basic concepts of CPR. Health care personnel had greater difficulty in recognizing the types of CPR, the importance of identifying defibrillable cardiac rhythms lies in the fact that it favors the survival of the victim with CPR.

Regarding the level of knowledge of chest compression in CPR, a medium level was obtained with 67%. There is discrepancy with the study done in Quito by Dr. Cynthia Cabrera Jurado, Dr. Christopher Cedillo Carrión where knowledge was unsatisfactory. (51) There is concordance in the study done by Indira Gisella Reyes Moran where it was found that the majority of health personnel have a medium level with 46.5% and low with 31.4%.(14) CPR guidelines prioritize chest compressions over ventilation, since once CRA is identified, chest compressions should be started soon, thus reducing ischemia that leads to damage to important organs. For this reason, a medium level of knowledge of the chest compression technique may present shortcomings in the practice of these techniques and trigger a series of events at the circulatory level such as ischemia, which leads to damage to target organs and ends in a poor prognosis for the patient and even death.

In this study, in relation to the variable on airway management in CPR, it was found that the majority had a medium level of knowledge with 56%. There is concordance in the study done by Indira Gisella Reyes Moran where 64% have a medium level and 36% a low level. (14) The maneuvers performed to open the airway depend on the clinical condition of the patient. It is important to rule out cervical spine trauma before performing any movement on the victim, since when there is cervical injury, any movement, including the forehead-chin maneuver, may worsen the patient's condition due to spinal cord injury.

In relation to the variable on ventilation in CPR, it was found that the majority of the personnel have a high level of knowledge with 55%. There is a discrepancy with the study done by Indira Gisella Reyes Moran in relation to the level of knowledge of ventilation in CPR, with the majority of health personnel having a low level of 58.1% and a medium level of 34.9%. (14) The function of rescue ventilation is to allow the spontaneous breathing of the patient with CPR to be replaced. Therefore, it is important to perform the ventilation technique correctly. Often, due to lack of knowledge of the proper application of ventilation, ventilation is prioritized over chest compression, so that more time is spent on ventilation and good results are not achieved.

In relation to the variable on early defibrillation, it was found that most of the personnel have a high level with 65%, where there was difficulty in recognizing defibrillable cardiac rhythms. The timely defibrillation, allows the reversal of CPR along with cardiac compressions, increasing the survival of the victim in CPR. There is discrepancy with the study conducted by Dr. Cynthia Cabrera Jurado, Dr. Christopher Cedillo Carrión "few successes were obtained in its entirety and it was observed that it is easier for participants to recognize an asystole than a VF or SVT, and despite knowing what rhythm it is, they do not know whether to defibrillate or not, which is extremely alarming because if we do not know one of the most important steps to follow all the schematic management that should be done will not work, ending in the death of the patient" (51). (51)

And finally, regarding the variable on the administration of drugs, it was found that most of them have an average knowledge with 57%. There is a discrepancy in the study conducted by Dr. Cynthia Cabrera Jurado, Dr. Christopher Cedillo Carrión, regarding the assessment of the drug of choice and the dose to be administered in the case of ventricular fibrillation that does not respond to defibrillation, where 60% responded incorrectly. (51) Lack of information about the drugs used, the dose and route of administration, survival along with patient prognosis can be compromised by inappropriate drug use. Many of the drugs used have a long half-life, such as vasopressin, so the vasopressor effect persists in the post-resuscitation period compromising ventricular function. On the other hand, adrenaline increases the recovery of spontaneous circulation (ROSC), but not survival to discharge, in addition to a worse long-term neurological survival.

One of our objectives was to evaluate the level of knowledge and relate it to years of experience in which we were able to observe that there is no statistically significant difference. There is agreement with the study conducted in Mexico by Balcazar showed that 89.34% of health personnel presented an unsatisfactory level of knowledge "thus exposing that there are very serious deficiencies in the knowledge of cardiopulmonary resuscitation, and that the years of experience and the ability in resuscitation are not associated with the level of knowledge". (16) As in the Tanzanian study, the level of knowledge was found to decrease over the years, but this was not significant. (78). There is a discrepancy with the study carried out in Spain by Peláez where it was observed that 76.9% of the participants know CPR and this knowledge of CPR is directly related to the years of work experience. (15)

CHAPTER V

5. CONCLUSIONS AND RECOMMENDATIONS

5.6. CONCLUSION

• The training on basic and advanced cardiopulmonary resuscitation in public institutions has been the responsibility of each of the professionals since none of these health institutions provide the facility to do them, so in our research it was found that medical professionals who were trained by their own means during the last 3 years have a high and medium knowledge in equal percentage and a low percentage has not been trained.

• It is very important to mention that in the time of study to become professionals do not give us a basic subject such as first aid to have a broader knowledge to perform this action so that professionals have to be trained by their own means to have more knowledge in the workplace, as we can find countless cardiorespiratory arrest throughout our professional life, which indicates the importance of being prepared in case of presenting an arrest and to handle it in the most appropriate way, since not doing so we have a high lethality.

• The level of knowledge of CPR of the professional health personnel of the emergency department of the Hospital Sagrado Corazón de Jesús in the identification of cardiorespiratory arrest is high, but they are deficient in recognizing the chain of intrahospital survival and the types of cardiorespiratory arrest.

• The staff knows the main cause of airway obstruction in CRA and the patency maneuver without cervical injury, but there is a lack of knowledge about airway patency in patients with cervical injury.

• Knowledge in ventilation is high, if they know about the correct technique of applying mouth to mouth breathing, but they have deficiencies in recognizing the duration of each ventilation and the number of ventilations per minute with the advanced ventilation device (Ambu).

• Knowledge in the application of chest compressions is average. They know the application of cardiac massage, the frequency of compressions in adults and the characteristics of high quality CPR,

but they fail to recognise the relationship between compression
and the position that the pregnant woman should have to decrease the
aortocaval pressure in CPR.

• Knowledge of early defibrillation is high. They know the defibrillation technique, but they are deficient in recognizing the cases in which defibrillation should be performed.

• The knowledge of drug administration is average, they know which drug to use, but they have shortcomings in the dose used and the route of administration.

• The knowledge of basic and advanced cardiopulmonary resuscitation of the resident doctors and nursing graduates in relation to their years of experience, the highest percentage have a high knowledge.

• It was concluded that years of experience does not prove that they have more knowledge as long as they have not been trained, since the AHA (American Heart Association) guidelines are updated from time to time.

5.7. RECOMMENDATIONS

After analyzing the results we obtained in our research, we can recommend:

- Promote ongoing training in basic and advanced CPR for all health personnel who are part of the emergency area.
- Hospitals should teach courses on basic and advanced CPR to all health personnel, especially in the emergency area, since we are exposed to patients with cardiopulmonary arrest every day.
- The Ministry of Public Health should demand compliance and renewal of courses on basic and advanced CPR, as well as verify their validity endorsed by authorized centers.
- Encourage drills in each emergency area to assess the deficiencies of each piece of equipment.
- It is recommended that protocols for the care of patients with respiratory arrest be drawn up to enable emergency service personnel to act appropriately, following the guidelines of the AHA.

CHAPTER VI

6. BIBLIOGRAPHY

7. BIBLIOGRAPHY

1. HEARTS: Technical package for the management of cardiovascular diseases in primary health care. Access to essential medicines and technologies. Washington, D.C.: Pan American Health Organization; 2019.

2. Dr.C. Idoris Cordero Escobar (2017) The teaching of cardiopulmonary and cerebral resuscitation. The teaching of cardiopulmonary and cerebral resuscitation: Anesthesiology and Resuscitation Service. Hermanos Ameijeiras Clinical Surgical Hospital. Havana, Cuba. CorHealth 2017 Oct-Dec;9(4):279-281.

3. López, A; Delgado, W; Barrios, I; Samudio, M; Torales, J. (2017). Knowledge of basic and advanced adult cardiopulmonary resuscitation of resident physicians of a tertiary hospital in Paraguay. Mem. Inst. Invest. Sci. Health. 15(1): 63-72. Available at: http://scielo.iics.una. py/pdf/iics/v15n1/ 1812-9528-iics-15-01-00063.pdf.

4. D. Mozaffarian, E.J. Benjamin, A.S. Go, D.K. Arnett, M.J. Blaha, M. Cushman, et al. Heart Disease and Stroke Statistics-2016 Update: A Report From the American Heart Association Circulation, 133 (4) (2016 Jan 26), pp. e38-e360

5. Aranzábal, G; Verástegui, A; Quiñones, D; Quintana, L; Vilchez, M. (2017). Factors associated with the level of knowledge in cardiopulmonary resuscitation in hospitals in Peru. Colombian Journal of Anesthesiology. 45(2); 114-121. Available at: http://www.sciencedirect. com/science/article/pii/S01203 34717 300047.

6. Aldo López-González I, Walter Delgado II, Iván Barrios III, Margarita Samudio IV, Julio T013lesV. (2017). Knowledge on basic and advanced adult cardiopulmonary resuscitation of resident physicians of a third level hospital in Paraguay. Mem. Inst. Investig. Sci. Health. 2017;15(1):63-72

7. Overlay panelRaúl J. GazmuriMD, PhD, FCCM. (2017) In-hospital cardiopulmonary resuscitation of the adult patientin-hospital cardiopulmonary resuscitation of the adult patient. Clinica Las Condes Medical Journal. Volume 28, Issue 2, March-April 2017, Pages 228-238

8. By Robert E. O'Connor, MD, MPH, University of Virginia School of Medicine Last Modified Mar. 2017.Cardiopulmonary Resuscitation (CPR) in Adults

9. Verónica Victoria Márquez Hernández, Laura Helena Antequera Raynal, Soporte vital básico: Basado en las recomendaciones ERC-2015.

10. Idoris Cordero Escobar, La enseñanza de la reanimación cardiopulmonar y cerebral, 2017.

11. Kaihula et al. 2018, Assessment of cardiopulmonary resuscitation knowledge and skills among healthcare providers at an urban tertiary referral hospital in Tanzania.

12. Dr. Cynthia Cabrera Jurado Dr. Christopher Cedillo Carrión. (2019) "level of knowledge on basic and advanced adult life support in members of surgical teams practicing in reference hospitals in the city of quito, multicenter study. february - march 2019" dissertation prior to obtaining the title specialist in anesthesiology, resuscitation and pain therapy. pontificia universidad católica del ecuador.

13. European Resuscitation Council Guidelines for Cardiopulmonary Resuscitation 2010.

14. WHO. (2018). Top 10 causes of death. Retrieved from http://www.who.int/es/news-room/fact-sheets/detail/the top-10-causes of-death.

15. Reyes Moran, I. G. (2017). Cybertesis UNMSM. Level of knowledge of the

healthprofessional ,   Retrieved from: http://cybertesis.unmsm.edu.pe/bitstream/handle/ cybertesis/5911/Reyes_mi.pdf?sequence=1.

16. Occupational Nursing. (2017). Level of knowledge and skills of cardiopulmonary resuscitation in workers: Retrieved from: NivelDeConocimientoYAptitudDeLaReanimacionCardio- 6279151%20(2).pdf.

17. Balcázar-Rincón LE, Mendoza-Solís LA, Ramírez-Alcántara YL. Cardiopulmonary resuscitation: level of knowledge among emergency department staff. Rev Esp Méd Quir 2015; 20:248-255.

18. American Heart Association. (2017). 2017 summary statistics. Heart disease and stroke: Retrieved from: https: //professional.heart.org/idc/groups/ahamah- public/@wcm/@sop/@smd/ documents/downloadable/ucm_491392.pdf.

19. López, A; Delgado, W; Barrios, I; Samudio, M; Torales, J. (2017). Knowledge of basic and advanced adult cardiopulmonary resuscitation of resident physicians of a tertiary hospital in Paraguay. Mem. Inst. Invest. Sci. Health. 15(1): 63-72. Available at: http://scielo.iics.una. py/pdf/iics/v15n1/ 1812-9528-iics-15-01-00063.pdf.

20. CarmenEscribaMendoza,   Wilber   Sulcabarrón,KNOWLEDGEAND SKILLSINBASICCPRMANAGEMENTIN NURSING PROFESSIONALS IN THEHEALTHCENTER.

21. Ricardo Arrabal Sánchez. Thoracic Surgeon. Thoracic Surgery Service. Regional Hospital of Malaga, CARDIORRESPIRATORY ARREST,2016

22. David F Gaieski, MD, Mark E Mikkelsen, MD, MSCE. Definition, classification, etiology, and pathophysiology of shock in adults. UpToDate 2016

23. Dr. Pedro E. Nodal Leyva1 Dr. Juan G. López Héctor2 and Dr. Gerardo de La Llera Domínguez3. Cardiorespiratory arrest. Rev. Cubana Cir.2015

24. Balaguer-Gargallo M, Cambra-Lasaosa FJ, Cañadas-Palazón S, Mayol-Canals L, Castellarnau-Figueras E, De-Francisco-Prófumo A, et al. Suport vital bàsic i avançat pediatr 2015. Pediatr catalana. 2016; 76(4):157-61.

25. Jara, Y. (March 11, 2016). BASIC PEDIATRIC CARDIOPULMONARY RESUSCITATION MANEUVERS. Asociación Española de Pediatría,159-172. Obtenidode http://www.aeped.es/sites/default/files/documentos/capitulo_5_0.pdf

26. Duff JP, Topjian A, Be rg MD, et al. 2018 American Heart Association focused update on pediatric advanced life support: an update to the American Heart Association guidelines for cardiopulmonary resuscitation and emergency cardiovascular care. Circulation. 2018; 138(23): e731- e739. PMID: 30571264 pubmed.ncbi.nlm.nih.gov/30571264/.

27. Carolina Tamayo Munera Diego Alejandro Muñoz Rincón Pediatrician Physician Subsp. in Intensive Care Critical Care Emergency Physician Pediatric Advanced Cardiopulmonary Resuscitation © Hospital Pablo Tobón Uribe Medellín - Colombia All Rights Reserved April 2016 - Third Edition

28. Abel Martínez Mejías Servicio de Pediatría Consorci Sanitari de Terrassa DIAGNOSTIC AND THERAPEUTIC PROTOCOLS IN PEDIATRIC EMERGENCIES Sociedad Española de Urgencias de Pediatría (SEUP), 3rd Edition, 2019

29. López Herce, J., Rodríguez Nuñez, A., Carrillo Alvárez, Á., Zeballos Sarrato, G., Martínez Fernández, C., & Calvo Macías, C. (2017). Expert recommendations on pediatric and neonatal cardiopulmonary resuscitation trolley and backpack material. Annals of Pediatrics, 173.e1-173.e7.

30.

31. Rojas L, Aizman A, Arab JP, Utili F, Andresen M. Basic cardiopulmonary resuscitation: theoretical knowledge, practical performance and effectiveness of maneuvers in general practitioners. Rev Med Chile. 2012;140(1):73-7

32. Sastre Carrera MJ, García LM, Bordel Nieto F, López-Herce Cid J, Carrillo Álvarez A, Benítez Robredo MT, et al. Teaching basic cardiopulmonary resuscitation in the general population. Aten Primaria. 2004; 34(8):408-13.

33. Overlay panel Raúl J. GazmuriMD, PhD, FCCM. (2017) In-hospital cardiopulmonary resuscitation of the adult patientin-hospital cardiopulmonary resuscitation of the adult patient. Clinica Las Condes Medical Journal. Volume 28, Issue 2, March-April 2017, Pages 228-238

34. J. Tirkkonen, H. Hellevuo, K.T. Olkkola, S. Hoppu Aetiology of in-hospital cardiac arrest on general wards Resuscitation, 107 (2016 Oct), pp. 19-24, 10.1016/j.resuscitation.2016.07.007 Epub; %2016 Aug 1.:19-24.

35. Indira Gisella Reyes Moran. (2016) Level of knowledge of the health professional on basic cardiopulmonary resuscitation in the Emergency Service of the National Maternal Perinatal Institute Lima - Peru 2016.

36. López-González A, Delgado W, Barrios I, Samudio M, Torales J. Knowledge of basic and advanced cardiopulmonary resuscitation in adult residents of a tertiary hospital in Paraguay. Mem. Inst. Investig. Sci. Health. 2017; 15(1): 63-72

37. S.M. Perman, E. Stanton, J. Soar, R.A. Berg, M.W. Donnino, M.E. Mikkelsen, et al. Donnino, M.E. Mikkelsen, et al. Location of In-Hospital Cardiac Arrest in the United States-Variability in Event Rate and Outcomes J Am Heart Assoc, 5 (10) (2016 Sep 29), p. e003638

38. L.W. Andersen, A. Granfeldt, C.W. Callaway, S.M. Bradley, J. Soar, J.P. Nolan, et al. Callaway, S.M. Bradley, J. Soar, J.P. Nolan, et al. Association Between Tracheal Intubation During Adult In- Hospital Cardiac Arrest and Survival JAMA, 317 (5) (2017 Feb 7), pp. 494- 506.

39. S.C. Brooks, M.L. Anderson, E. Bruder, M.R. Daya, A. Gaffney, C.W. Otto, et al. Otto, et al. Part 6: Alternative Techniques and Ancillary Devices for Cardiopulmonary Resuscitation: 2015 American Heart Association Guidelines Update for Cardiopulmonary Resuscitation and Emergency Cardiovascular Care Circulation, 132 (18 Suppl 2) (2015 Nov 3), pp. S436-S443

40. H. Wagner, C.J. Terkelsen, H. Friberg, J. Harnek, K. Kern, J.F. Lassen, et al. Cardiac arrest in the catheterisation laboratory: a 5-year experience of using mechanical chest compressions to facilitate PCI during prolonged resuscitation efforts Resuscitation, 81 (4) (2010 Apr), pp. 383-387.

41. J. Blumenstein, J. Leick, C. Liebetrau, J. Kempfert, L. Gaede, S. Gross, et al. Extracorporeal life support in cardiovascular patients with observed refractory in-hospital cardiac arrest is associated with favourable short and long-term outcomes: A propensity-matched analysis Eur Heart J Acute Cardiovasc Care, 5 (7) (2016 Nov), pp. 13-22.

42. R.J. Gazmuri, D.J. Patel, R. Stevens, S. Smith Circulatory collapse, right ventricular dilatation, and alveolar dead space: A triad for the rapid diagnosis of massive pulmonary embolism Am J Emerg Med, 16 (2016 Dec 16), p. 10.

43. P.A. Meaney, B.J. Bobrow, M.E. Mancini, J. Christenson, A.R. de Caen, F. Bhanji, et al. Cardiopulmonary resuscitation quality: improving cardiac resuscitation outcomes both inside and outside the hospital: a consensus statement from the American heart association Circulation, 128 (4) (2013 Jul 23), pp. 417-435.

44. W. Tang, M.H. Weil, R.J. Gazmuri, S. Sun, C. Duggal, J. Bisera Pulmonary ventilation/perfusion defects induced by epinephrine during cardiopulmonary resuscitation Circulation, 84 (1991), pp. 2101-2107

45. R.J. Gazmuri, M. von Plant a, M.H. Weil, E.C. Rackow Cardiac effects of carbon dioxide-consuming and carbon dioxide- generating buffers during cardiopulmonary resuscitation J Am Coll Cardiol, 15 (1990), pp. 482-490

46. R.W. Neumar, C.W. Otto, M.S. Link, S.L. Kronick, M. Shuster, C.W. Callaway, et al. Callaway, et al. Part 8: adult advanced cardiovascular life support: 2010 American Heart Association Guidelines for Cardiopulmonary Resuscitation and Emergency Cardiovascular Care Circulation, 122 (18 Suppl 3) (2010 Nov 2), pp. S729-S767

47. A.S. Chopra, N. Wong, C.P. Ziegler, L.J. Morrison Systematic review and meta-analysis of hemodynamic-directed feedback during cardiopulmonary resuscitation in cardiac arrest Resuscitation, 101 (2016 Apr), pp. 102-107,

48. R.J. Gazmuri, C.L. Kaufman, A. Baetiong, J. Radhakrishnan Ventricular Fibrillation Waveform Changes during Controlled Coronary Perfusion Using Extracorporeal Circulation in a Swine Model PLoS One, 11 (8) (2016 Aug 18), p. e0161166.

49. Albuerne AM. Cardiopulmonary resuscitation of the pregnant woman in the hospital environment. NPunto [Internet]. 2019 [cited 2020 Mar 18]; 2(15). Available from: https://www.npunto.es/revista/15/reanimacion- cardiopulmonar-de-la-gestante-en-el-medio-hospitalario.

50. Alonso T. Management of CRP in Pregnant Women. [Internet]. 2016. [cited 2016 Sep 262019   ]. Available at: http://congresoenfermeria.com/libros/2016/sala7/6091.pdf

51. Valdés O. Cardiopulmonary-cerebral resuscitation in the obstetric patient. Rev Cub Med Int Emerg. 2017; 16:54-88

52. Jeejeebhoy FM, Zelop CM, Lipman S, Carvalho B, Joglar J, Mhyre JM, et al. Cardiac Arrest in Pregnancy: A Scientific Statement from the American Heart Association. Circulation. 2015; 132(18):1747-73.

53. Ojeda JJ, Rodríguez M, Estpa JL, Piña CN, Cabeza BL. Physiological changes during pregnancy. Its importance for the anesthesiologist. MediSur. 2011; 9(5) 484-91.

54. Purizaca M. Physiological modifications in pregnancy. Rev Peru Ginecol y Obstet.2010; 56(1):57-69.

55. Magaldi M, Carretero J, Caballero Á, Matute EC. Cardiopulmonary resuscitation in the pregnant woman. Update according to 2015 guidelines. [Internet]. Societat Catalana D'Anestesiologia I Reanimació; 2016. [cited 2020 Feb 11]. Available from: http://www.academia.cat/files/204- 5509-FITXER/RCPGestante.pdf.

56. Calvo J. Particularities of cardiopulmonary resuscitation in the pregnant patient. Rev Med Cos Cen.2011; 68(596):115-19.

57. Sharan R, Madan A, Makkar V. Case report on effective cardiopulmonary resuscitation in a pregnant woman. Anesth Essays Res. 2016; 10(1):122.

58. Pueblas S, Marcovecchio M, Picech E, Laks J, Hernandez Y, Fernández F, et al. CPR and Pregnancy Protocol. [Internet]. Buenos Aires: 2016. [cited 2020 Feb   11].   Available   from: http://www.fasgo.org.ar/images/PROTOCOLO_DEL_MANEJO_DEL_PA RO_CARDIORRESPIRATORIO_EN_LA_MUJER_EMBARAZADA.pdf.

59. Monsieurs KRG, Nolan JP, Bossaert LL, Greif R, Maconochie IK, Nikolaou NI, et al. European Resuscitation Council Guidelines for Resuscitation 2015. Resuscitation. 2015; 95:1-80.
60. Sáenz ME, Vindas CA. Cardiac Arrest in Pregnancy. Rev Costarric Cardiol. 2014; 15(2):35-43.
61. GENERAL REGULATIONS TO THE ORGANIC LAW OF THE PUBLIC SERVICE Executive Decree 710 Official Gazette Supplement 418 of 01-Apr.-2011 Last modification: 28-Sep.-2018 Status: Amended. http://www.cpccs.gob.ec/wp-

INDEX OF ANNEXES

ANNEX:

BASIC/ADVANCED CPR) RECEIVED BY THE PROFESSIONAL STAFF OF THE HEALTH OF THE SACRED HEART OF JESUS HOSPITAL EMERGENCY AREA

"Q" DISTRIBUTION BY CORRECT AND INCORRECT QUESTION OF THE HEALTH PROFESSIONAL STAFF OF THE EMERGENCY AREA OF THE HOSPITAL SAGRADO CORAZON DE JESUS

"R" DISTRIBUTION ACCORDING TO THE LEVEL OF KNOWLEDGE ON CARDIOPULMONARY RESUSCITATION ACCORDING TO THE YEARS OF WORK EXPERIENCE OF THE HEALTH PERSONNEL OF THE EMERGENCY AREA OF THE HOSPITAL SAGRADO CORAZON DE JESUS

"S." PHOTOGRAPHS DURING THE SURVEYS

ANNEX A OPERATIONALIZATION OF THE VARIABLE

VARIABLE	CONCEPT DEFINITION UAL	DEFINITION OF OPERATION ONAL	DIMENSIONS	INDICATIONS	ESCALA DE MEDICION
Knowledge of basic and advanced cardiopulmonary resuscitation and advanced	Collected information on basic and advanced cardiopulmonary resuscitation that can help restore the vital functions in the face of cardiorespiratory arrest	Information available to the health staff of the area emergency area on cardiopulmonary resuscitation (CPR), which will allow you to apply them during will allow you to apply them during care of a patient who presents with cardiopulmonary arrest.	General: PCR Identification CPR Concept	Definition of Cardiac Arrest *Types of PCR Signs and Symptoms of Cardiac Arrest Definition of resuscitation Chain of Survival CPR Sequence * High quality CPR *RCPen	Ordinal scale *High *Medium *Low
			Management of chest compressions	Depth Time Frequency location Compression of compression	Ordinal scale *High *Medium *Low
			Airway Management	Cause of Airway Obstruction Method to permeabilize the airway airway with cervical problem Method to clear via cervical problem	Ordinal scale *High *Medium *Low
			RCO in Pediatric s	Compression/ventilation ratio on patients pediatric	

				CPR in Pregnant Women	Technique of cardiac massage at	
				Ventilation	Compression/Ventilation Ratio Time Technique	Ordinal scale *High *Medium *Low
				Automated external defibrillation	Technique *Application	Ordinal scale *High *Medium *Low
				Drugs used in Basic Life Support	Dose frequency *Viade administration	Ordinal scale *High *Medium *Low

Variable	Definition	Type of variable	Scale	Indicator
Sex	Male organic condition or female	qualitative	Male Female	percentage
Age	Time the person has lived in completed years, up to the time of the survey. data	quantitative	Years completed	average
Length of work experience	Time in the profession up to the date of collection of the data	Quantitative	Years of work experience	average

Participatin g in CPR maneuvers in real life situations	Witnessing and assisting a cardiac arrest	quantitative	Number of events	average
Participatio n in CPR trainings	Attended CPR training or courses in the last 3 years	quantitative	• Basic CPR • Advanced CPR • None	percentage
Professiona l is health	Usual activity of a person for which he/she has prepared himself/herself	qualitative	List of health professionals	percentage

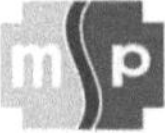

GUA⬛⬛⬛ ʹATE UNIVERSITY SURVEY
MEDICAL CAREER
DEGREE PROJECT: RESEARCH PROJECT

The present research project aims to obtain information about the knowledge of basic and advanced Cardiopulmonary Resuscitation that health personnel have in the emergency area of the Sacred Heart of Jesus Hospital in Quevedo, in the period between August-September 2020. I thank you in advance for your kind collaboration for the achievement of the purposes of this work and request that your answers be as truthful and sincere as possible. The survey is individual, anonymous and confidential, since your answers will only be used for the research project.

INSTRUCTIONS
Fill in the blanks and circle the letter of the item you think is correct.

GENERAL DATA:
1.- Sex: Female ( ) Male ( ) 2.- Age:______(years)
3.- Profession: Doctor ( ) Nurse ( )
4.-Time of work experience:________________(years)
5.-Participation in CPR training in the last 3 years: Basic CPR ( ) Advanced CPR ( ) None ( )
6.-Have you participated in CPR manoeuvres in real situations: YES ( ) NO ( )
N° of times:____________________

1) It is considered cardiorespiratory arrest when there is:
a. Sudden cessation of heart function and breathing
b. Pale skin, cold sweats, and precordial pain
c. Loss of consciousness and decreased breathing
d. Central and peripheral cyanosis

2) What are the types of Cardiorespiratory Arrest?
a. Ventricular Fibrillation, Asystole and Pulseless Electrical Activity.
b. Myocardial ischemia or infarction
c. Cerebral vascular accident
d. None

3) Basic Cardiopulmonary Resuscitation is defined as:
a. A set of actions to restore respiratory function.
b. Perform chest compressions, to restore cardiac arrest.

c. A set of actions to restore cardiac and respiratory functions, preventing brain damage.
d. An unexpected, abrupt cessation of respiratory and circulatory functions.

4) What are the steps in the chain of survival?
a. Immediate recognition of cardiorespiratory arrest and activation of the response system - compressions - defibrillator - advanced life support - comprehensive care
b. Immediate recognition of cardiorespiratory arrest and activation of the response system - check airway - compressions - advanced life support - defibrillator - comprehensive care
c. Airway - compressions - ventilation - chin lift - call a lifeguard.
d. Airway - Compressions - ventilations - AED - Immediate recognition of cardiopulmonary arrest and activation of the response system

5) In order to provide high quality basic CPR   ,   according to the new new recommendations we should: (indicate the incorrect one)
a. Allow full chest decompression after each compression.
b. The depth of compressions should be at least 5 cm in adults.
c. Minimize interruptions in chest compressions.
d. Compress with a frequency of less than 100 cpm.

6) The frequency of chest compressions in the adult recommended by the American Heart Association (AHA) is:
a. Less than 100 per minute.
b. At least 100 per minute.
c. Between 100 to 120 per minute.
d. From 80 to 100

7) The depth of chest compressions in an adult should be:
a. At least 2 inches (5 centimeters).
b. 1 ½ inch (4 centimeters).
c. At least 3 inches (7 centimeters).
d. At least 4 inches (10 centimeters).

8) Cardiac massage in adults is performed with:
a. 2 hands on the lower half of the sternum
b. 1 hand on the lower half of the sternum
c. 2 fingers in the center of the thorax
d. 2 fingers on the lower half of the sternum

9) The ratio of chest compressions/ventilations in adults when there is a rescuer is:
a. 10/1
b. 30/1
c. 30/2
d. 15/2

10) In the case of pregnant women, during chest compressions, the priority is to remove the aortocaval pressure, which must be done:
a. Manual uterine shift to the left
b. Manual uterine shift to the right
c. Place the pregnant woman in the prone position.
d. Place the pregnant woman in the gynecological position.

11) The technique used for airway patency in a victim who has suffered whiplash is:
a. Forehead - chin maneuver
b. Mandibular traction" manoeuvre
c. Finger sweeping for foreign bodies
d. Neck hyperextension

12) The purpose of raising the jaw and placing the head in the sniffing position is:
A) Free the upper airway from soft tissue obstruction.
B) Facilitate the visualization of a possible foreign body.
C) Stimulates breathing.
D) Avoid aspiration of regurgitated gastric fluid.

13) After opening the airway and closing the nose of an unresponsive adult or child, which of the following describes the best way to deliver mouth-to-mouth breaths?
a. Make an airtight seal between the victim's mouth and the rescuer's mouth and give 2 breaths, checking that the chest rises.
b. Place your mouth over the victim's mouth and administer small amounts of air and try to prevent the chest from rising.
c. Place mouth over victim's mouth and administer 1 slow breath for approximately 5 seconds.
d. Place your mouth over the victim's mouth and give 5 slow breaths.

14) If ventilating during CPR with an advanced airway device (AMBU), the provider should administer:
a. 2 breaths every 6 seconds (20 breaths per minute)
b. 1 breath every 6 seconds (10 breaths per minute)
c. 1 breath every 2 seconds (30 breaths per minute)
d. 1 breath every second (60 breaths per minute)

15) What is the most reliable method of confirming and monitoring the correct location of an endotracheal tube?
a. 5-point auscultation.
b. Colorimetric Capnography
c. Capnography continues
d. Use of esophageal detectors.

16) Cases in which defibrillation is necessary:
a. Atrial tachycardia and AV block

b.   Pulseless ventricular tachycardia and ventricular fibrillation
c.   Pulseless electrical activity
d.   Atrial fibrillation and asystole

17) Which drug is appropriately given in pulseless electrical activity?
a.   Atropine 0.5 mg at 2-4 minute intervals
b.   Atropine 1 mg at 3 to 5 minute intervals
c.   Adrenaline 1 mg at 3 to 5 minute intervals
d.   none of the above

18) What is the ideal route of administration of Adrenaline during cardiac arrest?
a.   IV
b.   IM
c.   Intracardiac
d.   Subcutaneous
e.   none of the above

19) Which drug is not used in basic life support to revive a cardiac arrest?
a.   Atropine
b.   Adrenaline
c.   Amiodarone
d.   Vasopressin
e.   none of the above

20) The rate of cardiac compressions during a resuscitation of a 3-year-old child should be:
A)   100 per minute. A compression-to-ventilation ratio of 15:2 when a rescuer is present.
B)   100 per minute with a compression-to-ventilation ratio of 15:2 when two resuscitators are present.
C)   100 per minute with a compression-to-ventilation ratio of 30:2 when two resuscitators are present.
D)   100 per minute with a compression-to-ventilation ratio of 30:2 regardless of whether there are one or two resuscitators.

Thank you for your cooperation

ANNEX C

AUTHORIZATION TO CONDUCT SURVEYS

Quevedo, 25 Agosto del 2020

HOSPITAL SAGRADO CORAZON DE JESUS

QUEVEDO

AUTORIZACIÓN DE TRABAJO DE TITULACIÓN

Yo, Dr Cando Palma Alex Orlando por medio del presente certifico que con mucho gusto habemos de brindarle nuestra colaboración para que pueda llevar a cabo su investigación en la realización de encuestas en el área de emergencia del Hospital Sagrado Corazón de Jesus ,sobre el tema: **Nivel de conocimiento sobre reanimación cardiopulmonar básico y avanzado en el personal de salud** todos los profesionales de esa área estamos para ofrecerle la ayuda que ustedes necesitan.

Les deseo muchos éxitos en su investigación y confiamos que de la misma resulte una aportación valiosa para su proyecto.

DR: CANDO PALMA ALEX ORLANDO

JEFE DEL AREA DE EMERGENCIA

ANNEX D

CERTIFICATE OF REVIEW OF THE QUESTIONNAIRE

Quevedo, 23 de Agosto del 2020

HOSPITAL SAGRADO CORAZON DE JESUS

QUEVEDO

Por medio del presente certifico haber realizado la revisión de la encuesta para el trabajo de tesis: **Nivel de conocimiento sobre reanimación cardiopulmonar básico y avanzado en el personal de salud** del cual son autoras las señoritas **Nelly Gabriela Cedeño Zambrano y Jineth Catalina Rodríguez Ordoñez**, realizado en el área de emergencia del Hospital Sagrado Corazón de Jesús de Quevedo, del periodo de Agosto-Septiembre del presente año.

Se eligieron 20 de las 35 preguntas formuladas, puedo garantizar que la información suministrada es confiable pues se basa en evidencia científica y actualizada.

Dr. Wladimir Albán Andrade

Anestesiología, Reanimación y Terapia del Dolor

94

ANNEX E

CATEGORIZATION OF THE VARIABLE LEVEL OF KNOWLEDGE ABOUT CARDIOPULMONARY RESUSCITATION

The Gaussian bell was used to classify the CPR knowledge of the health care personnel in the emergency area (resident physicians and nursing graduates) and it was divided into 3 categories:
HIGH, MEDIUM AND LOW.

Number of questions: 20

Arithmetic average: 10
Standard deviation: 6

We set the values for a and b a = 10 - (6 x 0.75) = 5.4 $\approx$ 5

b = 10 + (6 x 0.75) = 14.54 $\approx$ 15

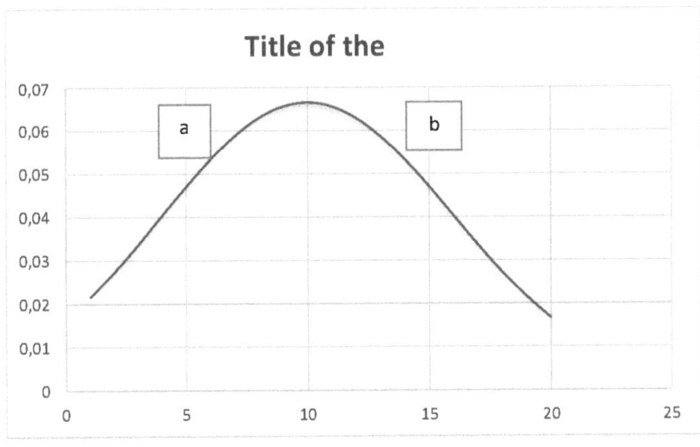

CATEGORIZATION OF THE DIMENSION LEVEL OF KNOWLEDGE ABOUT IDENTIFICATION OF SIGNS OF ARREST AND BASIC CONCEPTS ABOUT CPR

The Gaussian bell was used to classify the knowledge of emergency health personnel (resident physicians and nursing graduates) on the identification of CRP and basic concepts of RCO, divided into 3 categories: HIGH, MEDIUM, and LOW.

Number of questions: 5
Arithmetic average: 2.5
Standard deviation: 1.37

$$\overline{D.E} = \sqrt{1} \quad \frac{}{6} \quad (2,5-0)^2 + (2,5-1)^2 + (2,5-2)^2 + (2,5-3)^2$$

a = 2.5 - (0.75) x (1.37) = 1.47 ≈ 1

b= 2.5+ (0.75) x (1.37) = 3.57 ≈ 4

The values for a and b are set

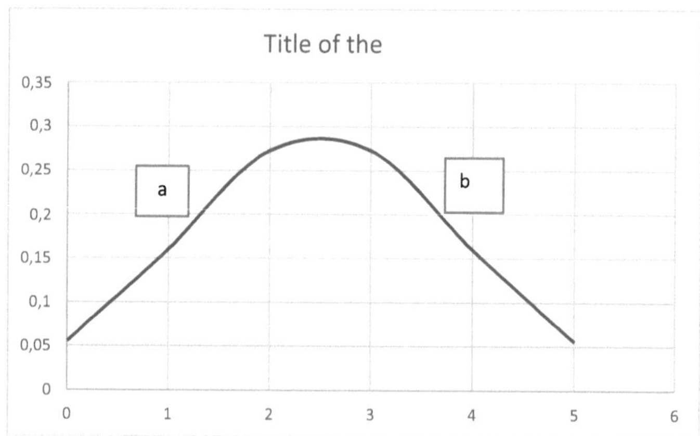

	PCR Identification					
PRE G NO.	P1	P2	P3	P4	P5	TOTAL
1	1	1	0	1	1	4
2	1	1	1	1	1	5
3	1	1	1	1	1	5
4	1	1	1	1	1	5
5	1	1	1	1	1	5
6	1	1	1	1	1	5
7	1	1	1	1	0	4
8	1	0	1	1	1	4
9	1	1	1	1	1	5
10	1	1	1	1	1	5
11	1	1	1	0	0	3
12	1	1	1	1	1	5
13	1	0	1	1	1	4
14	1	1	1	1	1	5
15	1	1	1	1	1	5
16	1	1	1	1	0	4
17	1	1	1	0	1	4
18	1	1	1	1	1	5
19	1	1	1	1	1	5
20	0	1	1	1	1	4
21	1	0	1	1	1	4
22	1	1	0	1	0	3
23	0	1	1	0	1	3
24	1	1	1	1	1	5
25	1	1	0	1	1	4
26	1	1	1	1	1	5
27	0	0	1	0	1	2
28	1	0	1	1	1	4
29	1	1	0	1	1	4
30	1	1	1	1	1	5
31	1	1	1	0	1	4
32	1	1	1	1	1	5
33	0	0	0	1	1	2
34	1	1	1	0	1	4
35	1	1	1	1	1	5
36	1	0	1	1	1	4
37	1	1	1	1	1	5
38	0	1	1	1	1	4
39	1	1	0	0	1	3
40	1	0	1	1	1	4
TOTAL	35	32	34	33	36	170

CATEGORIZATION OF THE DIMENSION LEVEL OF KNOWLEDGE ABOUT THORACIC COMPRESSION

The Gaussian bell was used to classify the knowledge of chest compressions of health personnel in the emergency area (resident physicians and nursing graduates) and it was divided into 3 categories: HIGH, MEDIUM AND LOW.

Number of questions: 4
Arithmetic average: 2
Standard deviation: 1

We set the values for a and b a = 2 - (0.75) x 1 = 1.25 $\approx$ 1

b = 2 + (0.75) x 1 = 2.75 $\approx$ 3

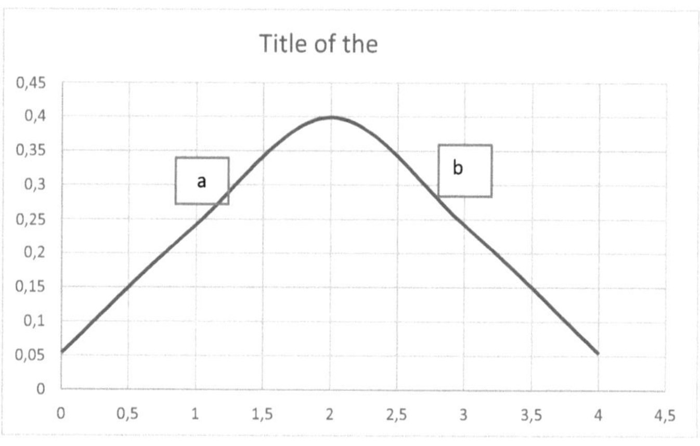

N°PREG	Thoracic compressions				TOTAL
	P6	P7	P8	P9	
1	0	1	1	1	3
2	1	1	0	1	3
3	1	0	1	1	3
4	0	1	1	0	2
5	1	0	1	1	3
6	1	1	0	1	3
7	0	1	1	1	3
8	1	1	1	1	4
9	1	0	1	0	2
10	1	1	0	1	3
11	0	1	1	1	3
12	1	1	1	1	4
13	1	1	0	1	3
14	1	1	1	0	3
15	1	1	1	1	4
16	1	1	1	1	4
17	0	1	0	1	2
18	1	1	1	1	4
19	1	0	1	1	3
20	1	1	1	1	4
21	1	1	1	0	3
22	1	1	1	1	4
23	1	1	0	0	2
24	0	1	1	1	3
25	1	1	1	1	4
26	1	1	0	1	3
27	1	1	1	1	4
28	0	0	1	1	2
29	1	1	0	0	2
30	1	1	1	1	4
31	1	0	1	1	3
32	1	1	1	1	4
33	0	0	1	1	2
34	1	1	0	1	3
35	1	0	1	0	2
36	0	1	1	1	3
37	1	1	1	1	4
38	1	1	0	1	3
39	1	0	0	1	2
40	1	1	1	1	4
TOTAL	31	31	29	33	124

CATEGORIZATION OF THE DIMENSION LEVEL OF KNOWLEDGE ABOUT AIRWAY MANAGEMENT

The Gaussian bell was used to classify the knowledge of airway management among health personnel in the emergency area (resident physicians and nursing graduates) and it was divided into 3 categories: HIGH, MEDIUM AND LOW.

Number of questions: 3
Arithmetic average: 1.5
Standard deviation: 1.12

We set the values for a and b a = 1,5 - (0,75) (1,12) = 0, 66 ≈ 1

b = 1,5 – (0,75) (1,12) = 2,34 ≈2

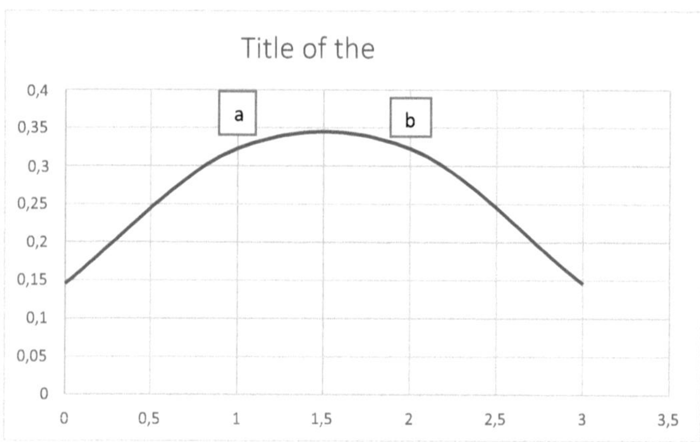

	Airway Management			TOTAL
PREG NO.	P10	P11	P12	TOTAL
1	1	1	1	3
2	0	1	1	2
3	0	1	1	2
4	0	1	0	1
5	1	1	0	2
6	0	1	1	2
7	0	1	0	1
8	0	1	1	2
9	0	1	0	1
10	1	1	1	3
11	1	1	1	3
12	0	1	1	2
13	0	1	1	2
14	1	1	1	3
15	1	1	1	3
16	0	1	1	2
17	0	1	1	2
18	1	0	1	2
19	0	1	1	2
20	0	1	1	2
21	1	0	0	1
22	0	1	1	2
23	0	1	0	1
24	0	1	1	2
25	1	0	1	2
26	0	0	1	1
27	0	1	0	1
28	0	1	1	2
29	1	1	1	3
30	1	1	1	3
31	1	1	1	3
32	0	0	0	0
33	1	0	1	2
34	0	1	1	2
35	1	1	0	2
36	0	1	1	2
37	0	1	0	1
38	1	1	1	3
39	0	1	1	2
40	0	1	1	2
TOTAL	16	35	31	82

CATEGORIZATION OF THE DIMENSION LEVEL OF KNOWLEDGE ABOUT VENTILATION

For the classification of the knowledge of ventilation of health personnel in the emergency area (resident physicians and nursing graduates), the Gaussian nursing bell was used and it was divided into 3 categories: HIGH, MEDIUM AND LOW.

Number of questions: 3
Arithmetic average: 1.5
Standard deviation: 1.12

We set the values for a and b a = 1,5 - (0,75) (1,12) = 0, 66 $\approx$ 1

b = 1,5 – (0,75) (1,12) = 2,34 $\approx$ 2

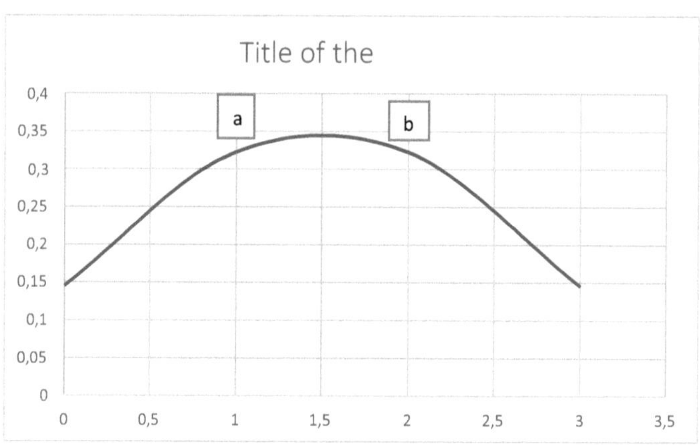

	Ventilation			
N°PREG	P13	P14	P15	TOTAL
1	0	1	1	2
2	1	0	1	2
3	1	0	1	2
4	1	0	0	1
5	1	1	1	3
6	1	1	1	3
7	1	1	1	3
8	1	1	1	3
9	1	0	1	2
10	1	1	1	3
11	1	1	0	2
12	1	1	1	3
13	1	1	1	3
14	1	1	1	3
15	1	0	1	2
16	1	1	1	3
17	1	1	1	3
18	1	1	1	3
19	1	0	1	2
20	1	0	1	2
21	0	1	1	2
22	1	1	1	3
23	1	1	1	3
24	1	1	1	3
25	1	1	1	3
26	1	0	0	1
27	0	1	1	2
28	1	1	1	3
29	1	1	1	3
30	1	1	1	3
31	0	1	1	2
32	1	0	1	2
33	1	1	1	3
34	0	1	0	1
35	1	1	1	3
36	1	1	1	3
37	1	0	1	2
38	1	1	1	3
39	0	0	1	1
40	1	1	0	2
TOTAL	34	30	36	100

CATEGORIZATION OF THE DIMENSION LEVEL OF KNOWLEDGE ABOUT EARLY DEFIBRILLATION

For the classification of knowledge of early defibrillation of health personnel in the emergency area (resident physicians and nursing graduates), the Gaussian nursing bell was used and it was divided into 3 categories: HIGH, MEDIUM AND LOW.

.

Number of questions: 2
Arithmetic average: 1
Standard deviation: 0.81

We set the values for a and b a = 1 - (0.75) (0.81) = 0.39 $\approx$ 0

b = 1 + (0,75) (0,81) = 1,6 $\approx$ 2

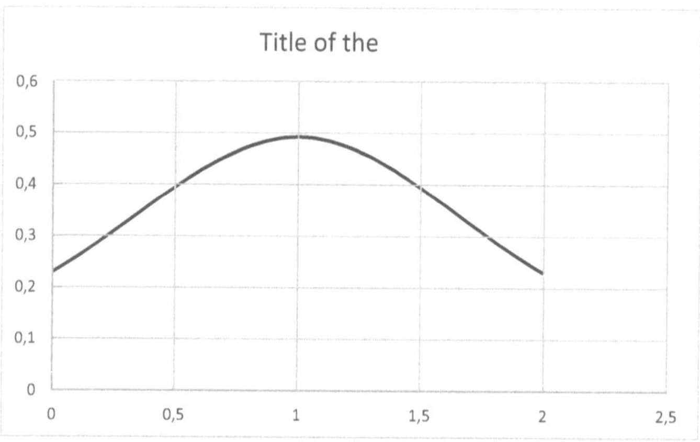

	Defibrillation		
N°PREG	P16	P17	TOTAL
1	1	1	2
2	1	0	1
3	1	1	2
4	1	1	2
5	0	1	1
6	1	0	1
7	1	1	2
8	1	0	1
9	0	1	1
10	1	1	2
11	1	1	2
12	1	0	1
13	1	1	2
14	1	1	2
15	1	1	2
16	0	1	1
17	1	0	1
18	1	1	2
19	1	1	2
20	1	1	2
21	1	1	2
22	1	1	2
23	1	1	2
24	1	0	1
25	1	1	2
26	1	1	2
27	1	1	2
28	1	1	2
29	1	1	2
30	0	1	1
31	0	1	1
32	0	1	1
33	1	0	1
34	1	1	2
35	1	1	2
36	1	0	1
37	1	1	2
38	1	1	2
39	1	1	2
40	1	1	2
TOTAL	34	33	67

CATEGORIZATION OF THE DIMENSION LEVEL OF KNOWLEDGE ABOUT DRUG ADMINISTRATION IN RCP

For the classification of knowledge on the administration of drugs in CPR among health personnel in the emergency area (resident physicians and nursing graduates), the Gaussian nursing bell was used and it was divided into 3 categories: HIGH, MEDIUM AND LOW.

Number of questions: 3
Arithmetic average: 1.5
Standard deviation: 1.2

We set the values for a and b a = 1,5 - (0,75) (1,12) = 0, 66 $\approx$ 1

b = 1,5 – (0,75) (1,12) = 2,34 $\approx$ 2

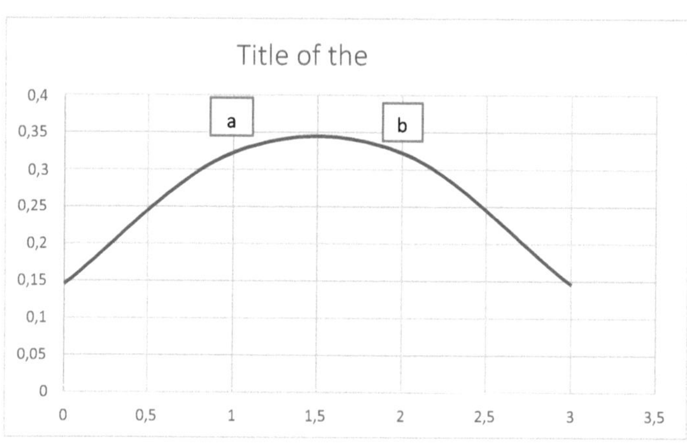

	Drugs in CPR			
N°PREG	P18	P19	P20	TOTAL
1	1	1	1	3
2	0	1	1	2
3	1	0	1	2
4	1	1	0	2
5	1	0	1	2
6	1	0	1	2
7	0	1	0	1
8	1	0	0	1
9	0	1	1	2
10	1	0	1	2
11	1	1	0	2
12	1	0	1	2
13	1	0	1	2
14	1	1	1	3
15	0	1	0	1
16	1	1	0	2
17	1	1	0	2
18	1	0	0	1
19	1	1	1	3
20	1	1	0	2
21	1	0	1	2
22	1	1	1	3
23	1	1	0	2
24	1	1	0	2
25	0	1	1	2
26	0	1	0	1
27	1	1	1	3
28	1	1	0	2
29	0	0	1	1
30	1	1	1	3
31	1	1	0	2
32	0	1	1	2
33	1	0	0	1
34	0	1	0	1
35	1	1	1	3
36	0	0	0	0
37	1	1	0	2
38	1	1	0	2
39	1	1	0	2
40	0	0	0	0
TOTAL	30	28	19	77

CODING LIST

Specific Data:

Knowledge of basic and advanced CPR:

1. Correct: 1 Incorrect: 0
2. Correct: 1 Incorrect: 0
3. Correct: 1 Incorrect: 0
4. Correct: 1 Incorrect: 0
5. Correct: 1 Incorrect: 0
6. Correct: 1 Incorrect: 0
7. Correct: 1 Incorrect: 0
8. Correct: 1 Incorrect: 0
9. Correct: 1 Incorrect: 0
10. Correct: 1 Incorrect: 0
11. Correct: 1 Incorrect: 0
12. Correct: 1 Incorrect: 0
13. Correct: 1 Incorrect: 0
14. Correct: 1 Incorrect: 0
15. Correct: 1 Incorrect: 0
16. Correct: 1 Incorrect: 0
17. Correct: 1 Incorrect: 0
18. Correct: 1 Incorrect: 0
19. Correct: 1 Incorrect: 0
20. Correct: 1 Incorrect: 0

MATRIX TABLE OF THE LEVEL OF KNOWLEDGE ON BASIC AND ADVANCED CARDIOPULMONARY RESUSCITATION OF THE HEALTH PERSONNEL OF THE EMERGENCY AREA OF THE HOSPITAL SAGRADO CORAZON DE JESUS, QUEVEDO

PCR Identification	Thoracic compressions	Airway Management	Ventilation	Defibrillation	Drugs in CPR	

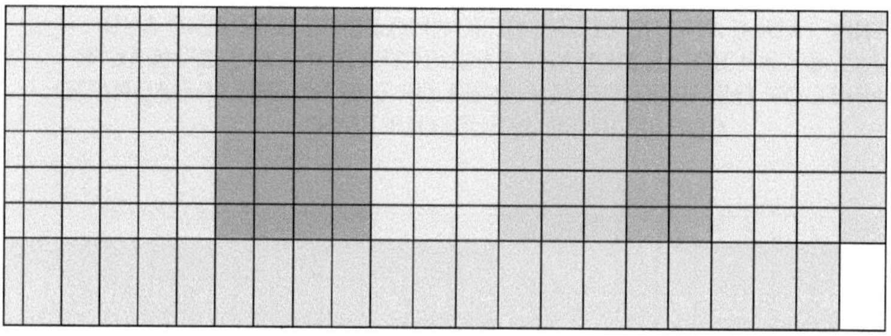

DISTRIBUTION BY AGE AND SEX OF HEALTH PERSONNEL IN THE EMERGENCY AREA OF THE HOSPITAL SAGRADO CORAZON DE JESUS IN THE CITY OF QUEVEDO - ECUADOR 2020

SEX / AGE	FEMALE		MALE		TOTAL	
	N°	%	N°	%	N°	%
27-37 years old	22	55	7	17,5	29	72,5
38-48 years old	5	12,5	1	2,5	6	15
49-59 years old	2	5	1	2,5	3	7,5
60 years and older	2	5	0	0	2	5
TOTAL	31	77,5	9	22,5	40	100

ANNEX N

DISTRIBUTION BY PROFESSION OF THE HEALTH PERSONNEL OF THE EMERGENCY AREA OF THE HOSPITAL SAGRADO CORAZON DE JESUS

PROFESSION	N°	%
General Emergency Resident Physician	25	62,5
Gynecological Emergency Resident Physician obstetric	5	12,5
General Emergency Nurse Practitioner	5	12,5
Licensed emergency gynecological nurse. obstetric	5	12,5
TOTAL	40	100

ANNEX Ñ

DISTRIBUTION BY TIME OF WORK EXPERIENCE OF THE HEALTH PERSONNEL OF THE EMERGENCY AREA OF THE HOSPITAL SAGRADO CORAZON DE JESUS

TIME OF EXPERIENCE LABOR	N°	%
1-5 years	22	55
6-10 years	7	17,5
11-15 years old	6	15
16-20 years old	3	7,5
More than 20 years	2	5
TOTAL	40	100

DISTRIBUTION BY CARDIOPULMONARY RESUSCITATION TRAINING RECEIVED IN
THE LAST 3 YEARS OF THE HEALTH PERSONNEL IN THE EMERGENCY AREA OF THE HOSPITAL SAGRADO CORAZON DE JESUS

TRAINING ABOUT CPR	N°	%
I RECEIVE	30	75
NO RECEIPT	10	25
TOTAL	40	100

DISTRIBUTION BY TYPE OF TRAINING (BASIC CPR / BASIC/ADVANCED CPR) RECEIVED BY THE HEALTH PERSONNEL OF THE EMERGENCY AREA OF THE HOSPITAL SAGRADO CORAZON DE JESUS

TYPE OF TRAINING	N°	%
BASIC	9	22%
BASIC AND ADVANCED	21	53%
NONE	10	25%
TOTAL	40	100%

DISTRIBUTION BY CORRECT AND INCORRECT QUESTION OF THE HEALTH PROFESSIONAL PERSONNEL OF THE EMERGENCY AREA OF THE HOSPITAL SAGRADO CORAZON DE JESUS

Questions	CORRECT O		INCORRECT		TOTAL	
	No	%	No	%	No	%
1	35	87,5	5	12,5	40	100
2	32	80	8	20	40	100
3	34	85	6	15	40	100
4	33	82,5	7	17,5	40	100
5	36	90	4	10	40	100
6	31	77,5	9	22,5	40	100
7	31	77,5	9	22,5	40	100
8	29	72,5	11	27,5	40	100
9	33	82,5	7	17,5	40	100
10	15	37,5	25	62,5	40	100
11	34	85	6	15	40	100
12	30	75	10	25	40	100
13	34	85	34	85	40	100
14	29	72,5	11	27,5	40	100
15	35	87,5	5	12,5	40	100
16	34	85	6	15	40	100
17	32	80	8	20	40	100
18	29	72,5	11	27,5	40	100
19	27	67,5	13	32,5	40	100
20	19	47,5	21	52,5	40	100

DISTRIBUTION ACCORDING TO THE LEVEL OF KNOWLEDGE ON CARDIOPULMONARY RESUSCITATION ACCORDING TO THE YEARS OF WORK EXPERIENCE OF THE HEALTH PERSONNEL OF THE EMERGENCY AREA OF THE HOSPITAL SAGRADO CORAZON DE JESUS

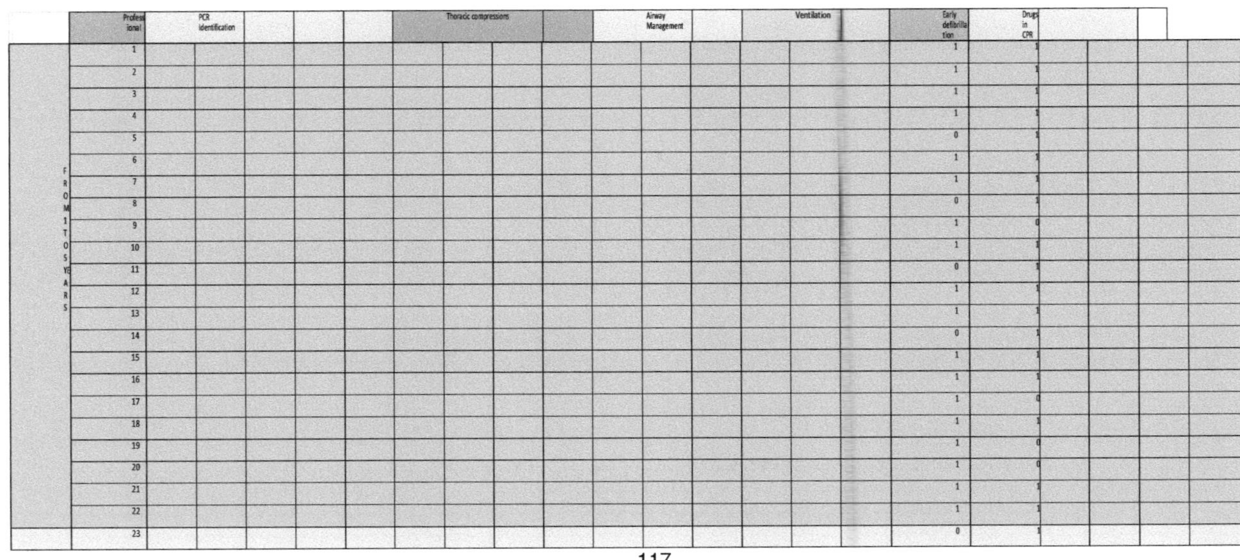

	Professional	PCR Identification	Thoracic compressions	Airway Management	Ventilation	Early defibrillation	Drugs in CPR
F	1					1	1
R	2					1	1
O	3					1	1
M	4					1	1
1	5					0	1
T	6					1	1
O	7					1	1
5	8					0	1
Y	9					1	0
E	10					1	1
A	11					0	1
R	12					1	1
S	13					1	1
	14					0	1
	15					1	1
	16					1	1
	17					1	0
	18					1	1
	19					1	0
	20					1	0
	21					1	1
	22					1	1
	23					0	1

Group	Row		
FROM 6 TO 10 YEARS OLD	24	1	0
	25	0	1
	26	1	1
	27	1	0
	28	1	0
	29	1	1
FROM 11 TO 15 YEARS OLD	30	1	1
	31	1	1
	32	1	1
	33	1	1
	34	1	1
	35	1	1
FROM 16 TO 20 YEARS OLD	36	1	1
	37	1	1
	38	1	1
OVER	39	1	0
	40	1	1

	Profes sional	corre ct	%
FROM 1 TO 5 YEARS	1	12	60
	2	14	70
	3	14	70
	4	15	75
	5	15	75
	6	17	85
	7	17	85
	8	16	80
	9	16	80
	10	14	70
	11	13	65
	12	16	80
	13	13	65
	14	16	80
	15	18	90
	16	15	75
	17	17	85
	18	17	85
	19	15	75
	20	15	75
	21	16	80
	22	19	95
FROM 6 TO 10 YEARS OLD	23	14	70
	24	11	55
	25	19	95
	26	13	65
	27	16	80
	28	14	70
	29	17	85
FROM 11 TO 15 YEARS OLD	30	14	70
	31	17	85
	32	17	85
	33	16	80
	34	17	85
	35	13	65
FROM 16 TO 20 YEARS OLD	36	13	65
	37	17	85
	38	15	75
OVER 20 YEARS OF EXPERIENCE	39	13	65
	40	16	80

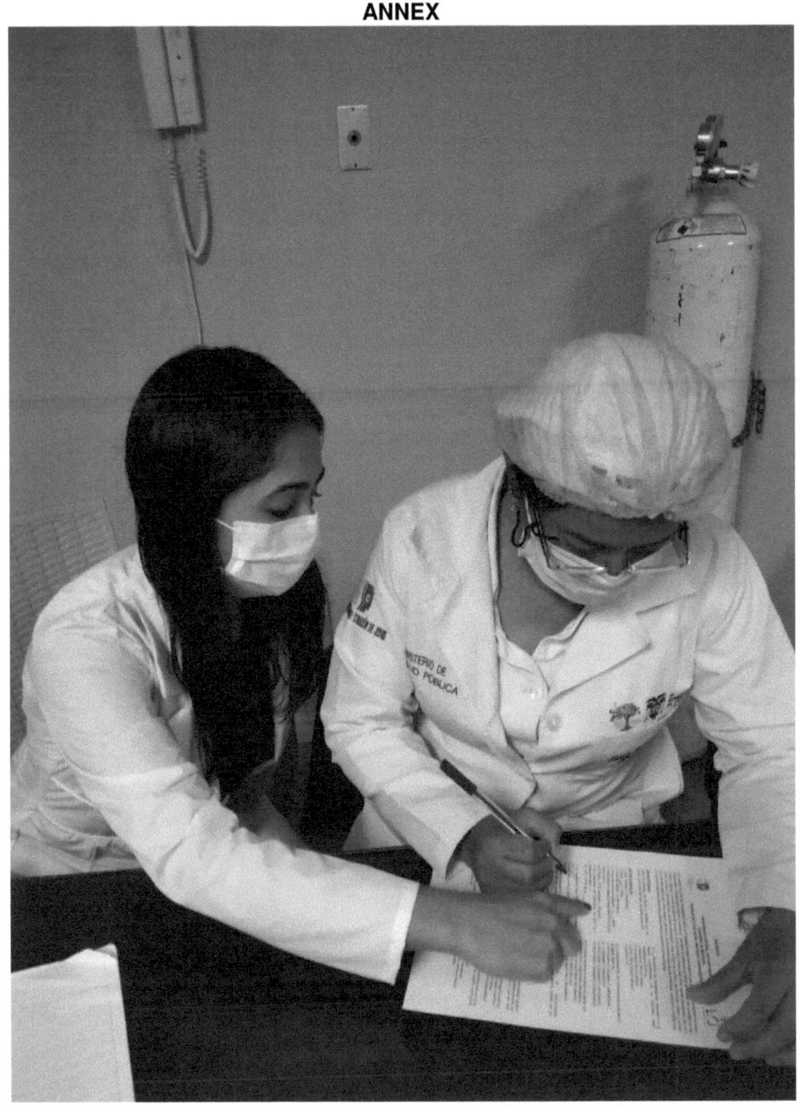

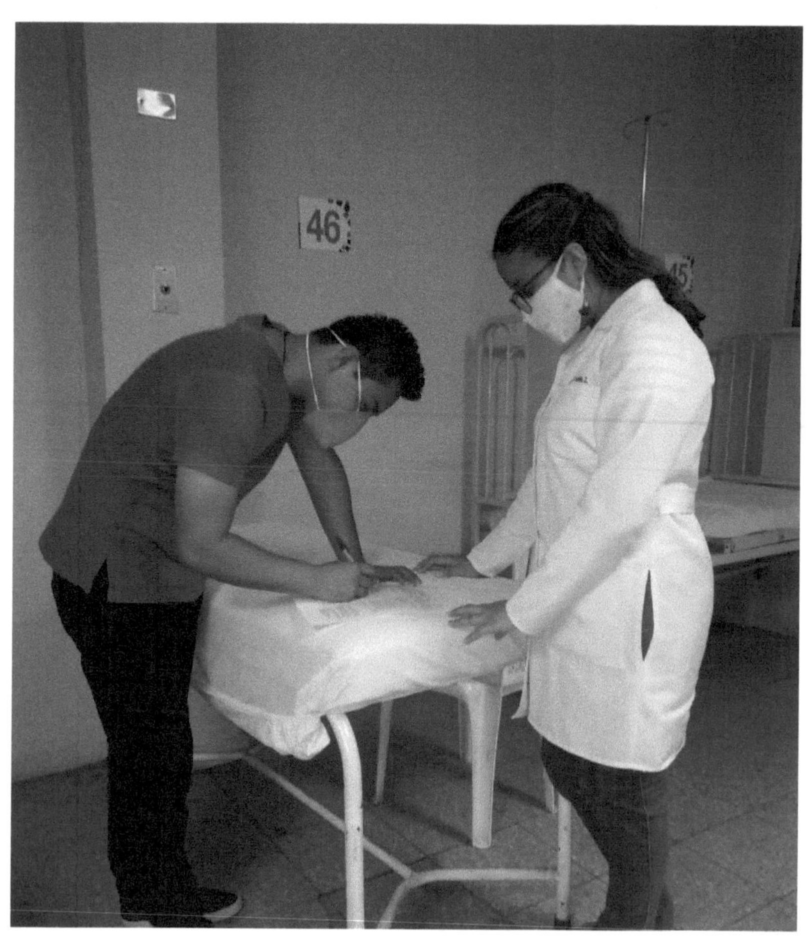

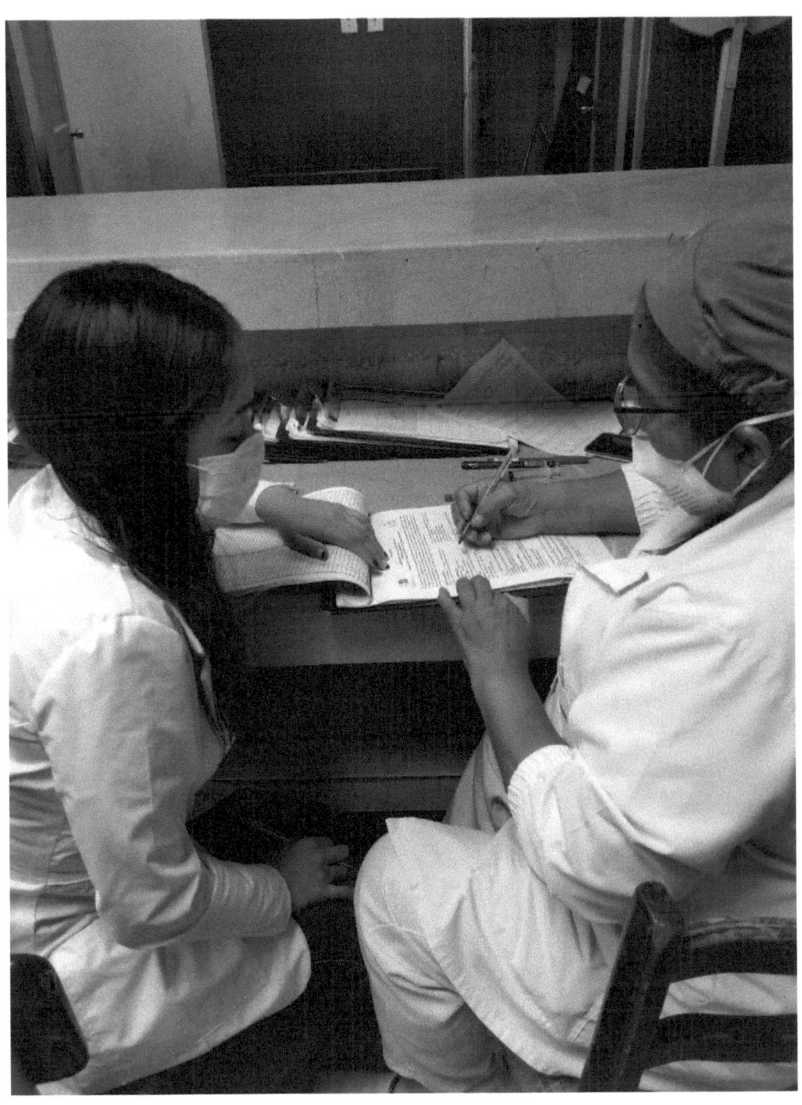

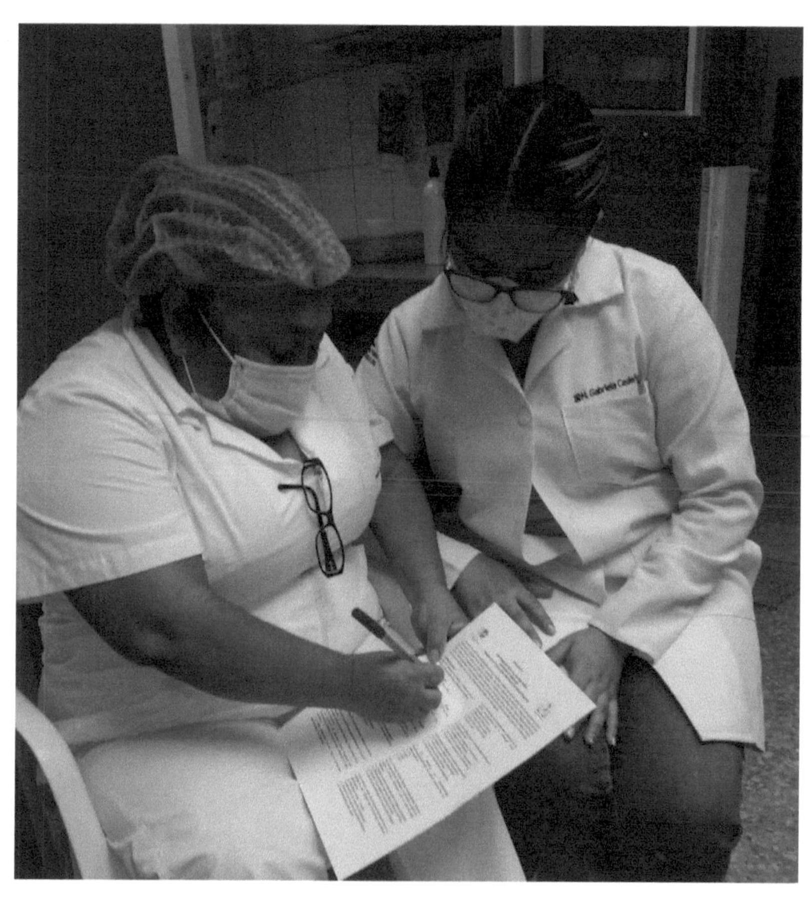

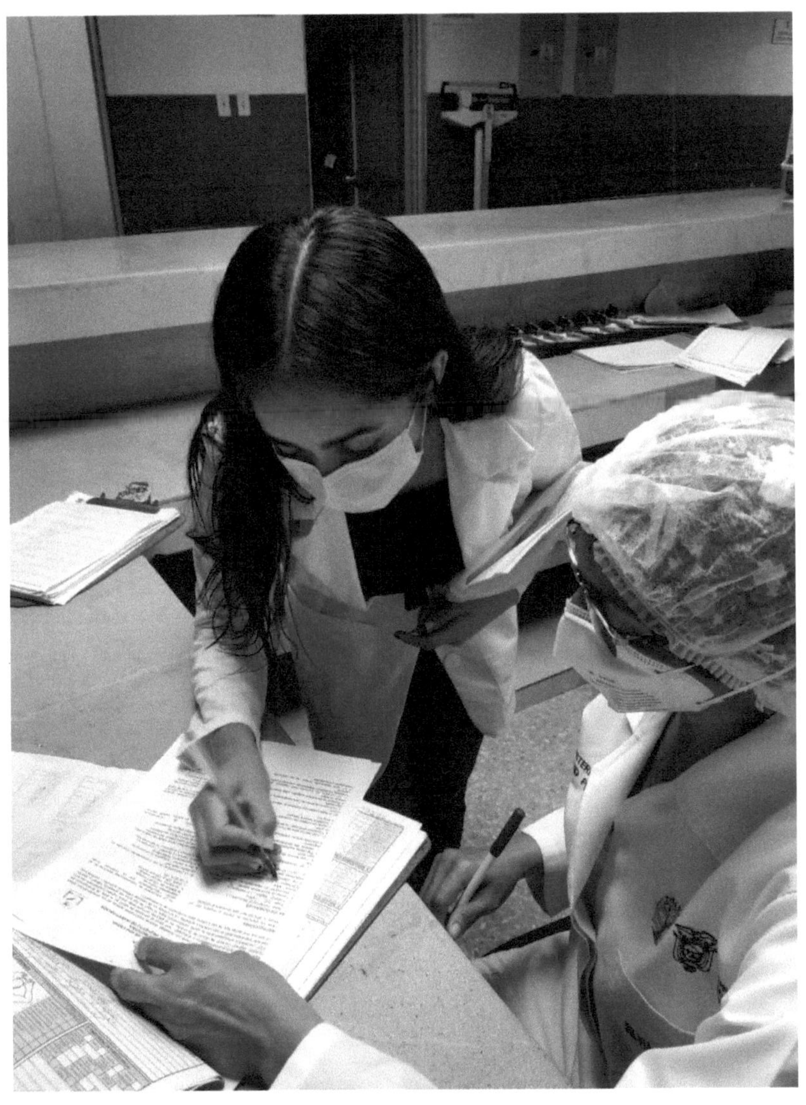

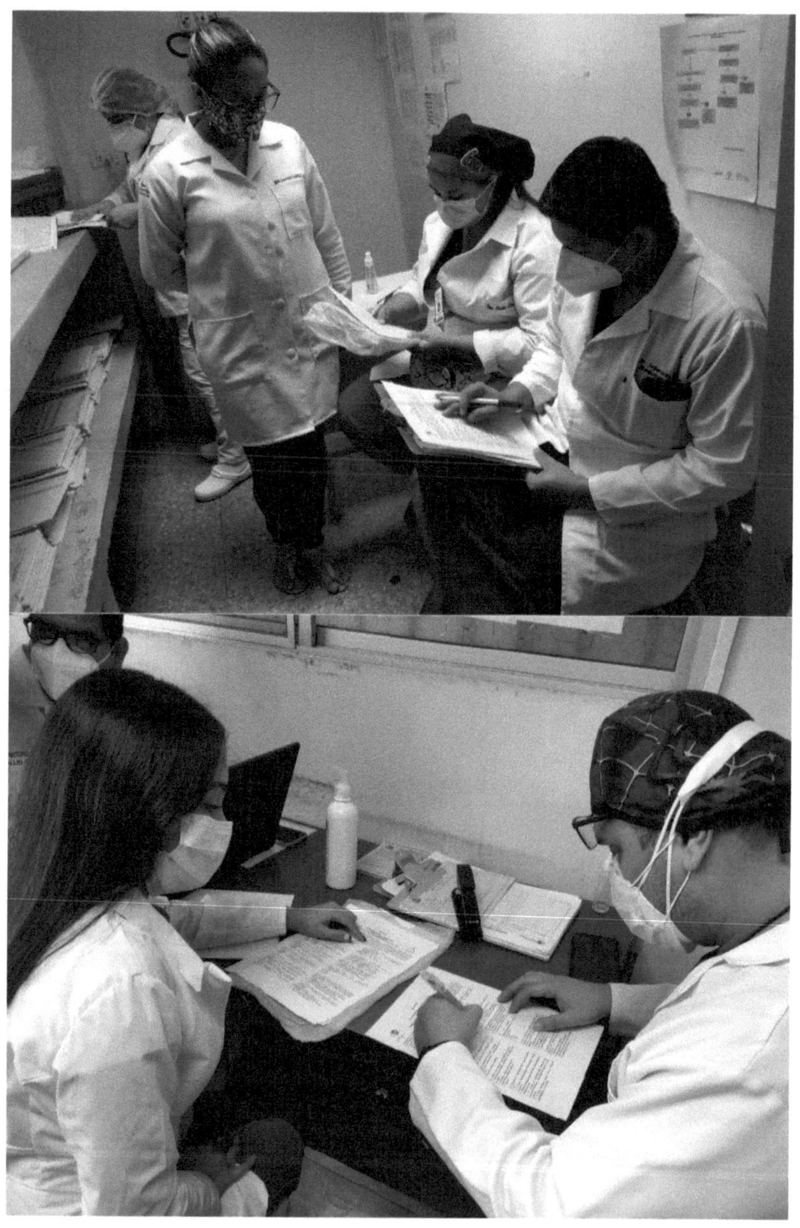

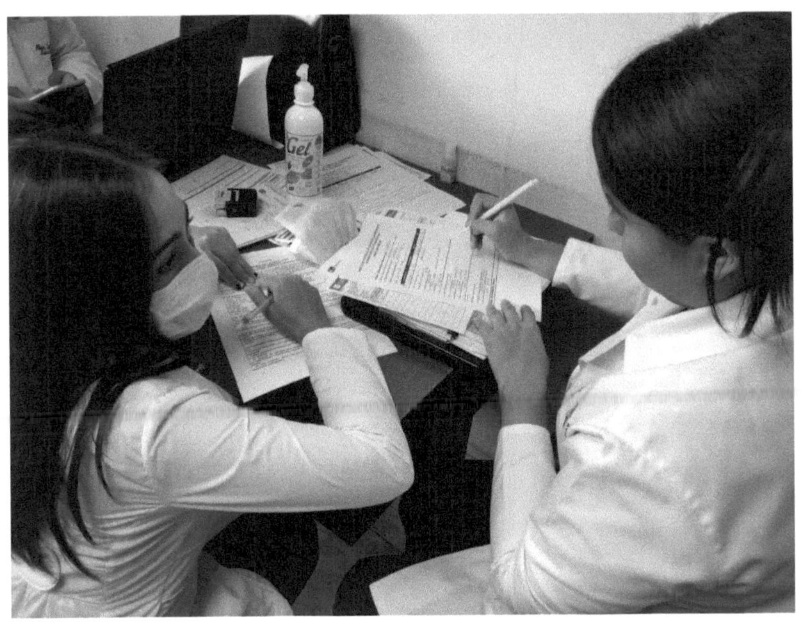

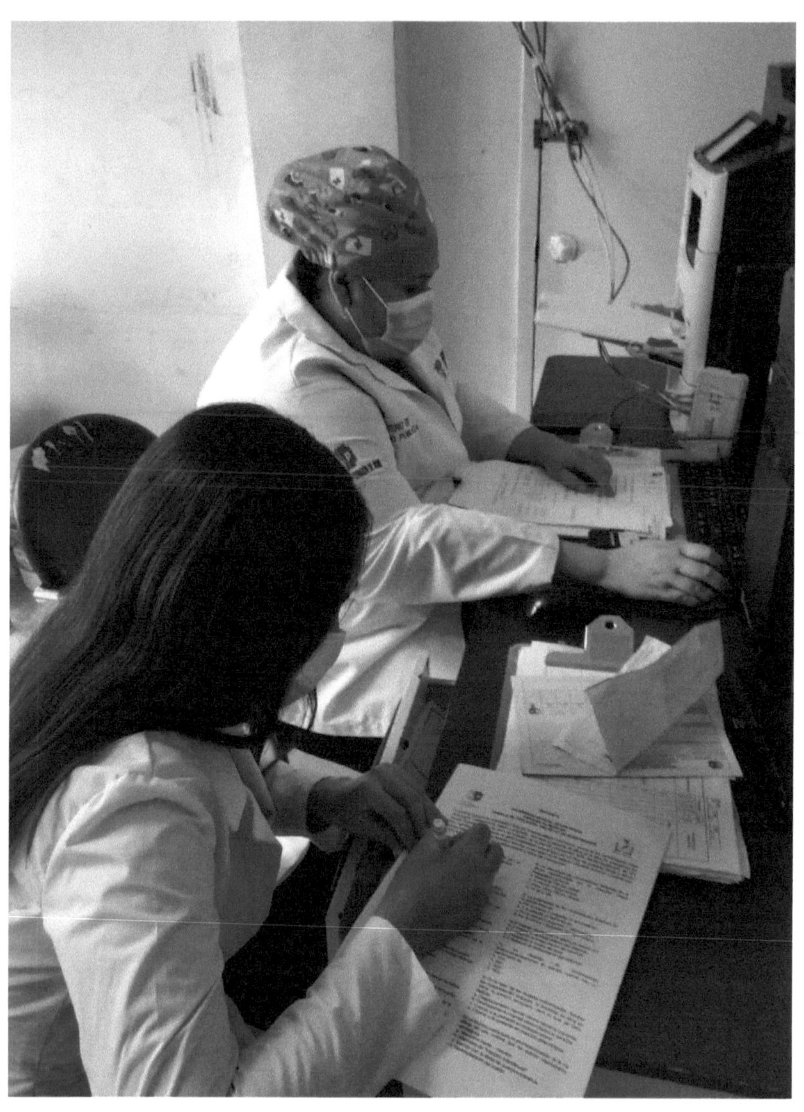

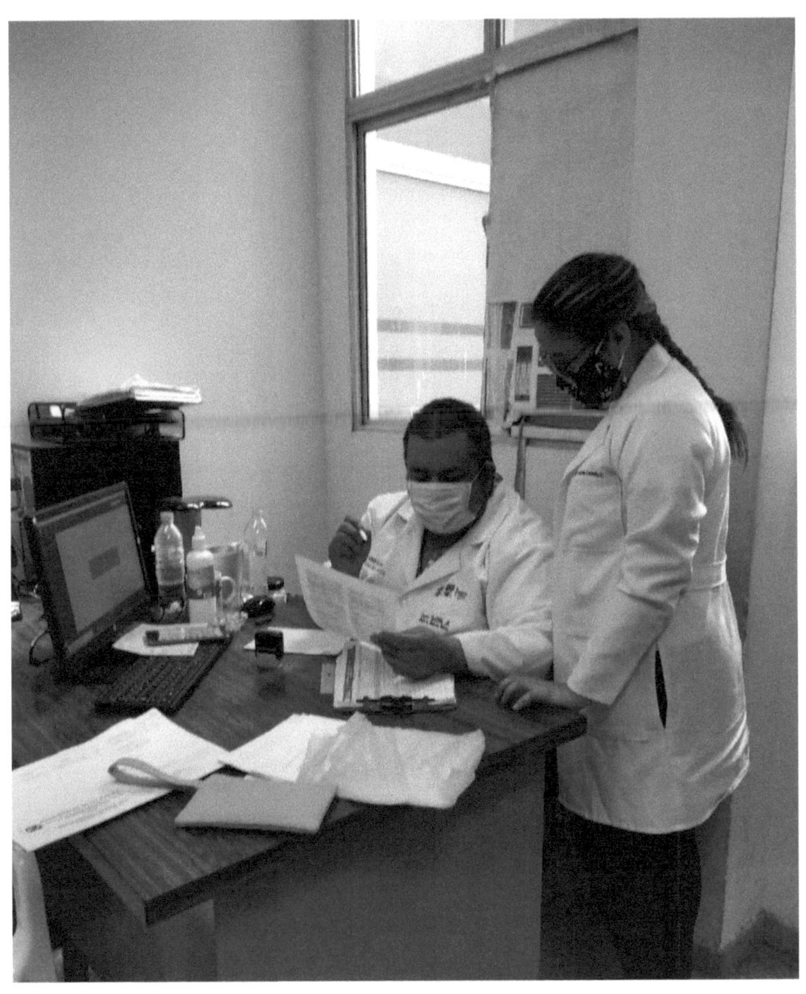

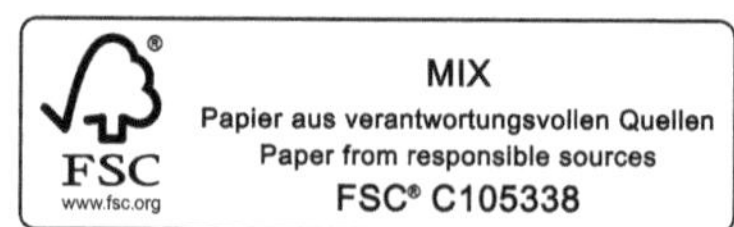

Printed by Books on Demand GmbH, Norderstedt / Germany